Marketing Strategies for Human and Social Service Agencies

The *Health Marketing Quarterly* series, William J. Winston, Editor:

- *Marketing the Group Practice: Practical Methods for the Health Care Practitioner*
- *Marketing for Mental Health Services*
- *Marketing Long-Term and Senior Care Services*
- *Innovations in Hospital Marketing*
- *Marketing Ambulatory Care Services*
- *Marketing Strategies for Human and Social Service Agencies*
- *Marketing Ambulatory Care Services*
- *Marketing Strategies for Human and Social Service Agencies*
- *Health Marketing and Consumer Satisfaction: A Guide to Basic Linkages*

ABOUT THE EDITOR

William J. Winston is Dean, School of Health Services Management, Golden Gate University, San Francisco, CA; Managing Associate, Professional Services Marketing Group, an Albany, CA based professional services marketing consulting firm; and senior editor for Marketing, The Haworth Press, Inc., New York, NY.

Marketing Strategies for Human and Social Service Agencies

William J. Winston
Editor

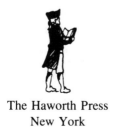

The Haworth Press
New York

Marketing Strategies for Human and Social Service Agencies has also been published as *Health Marketing Quarterly,* Volume 2, Number 4, Summer 1985.

The Haworth Press, Inc., 28 East 22 Street, New York, NY 10010

Library of Congress Cataloging in Publication Data
Main entry under title:

Marketing strategies for human and social service agencies.

Published also as Health marketing quarterly, v. 2, no. 4, summer 1985.
Includes bibliographies and index.
1. Social service—United States—Marketing—Addresses, essays, lectures. 2. Public relations—Social service—United States—Addresses, essays, lectures. I. Winston, William J. [DNLM: 1. Community Health Services. 2. Marketing of Health Services. 3. Social Work. W1 HE414D v. 2 no. 4/W74 M34567]
HV91.M288 1985   361'.0068'8   85-8534
ISBN 0-86656-355-5
ISBN 0-86656-468-3 (pbk.)

Marketing Strategies
for Human and Social Service Agencies

Health Marketing Quarterly
Volume 2, Number 4

CONTENTS

Preface

This issue completes the second year of the *Health Marketing Quarterly.* During the past two years, we have had the opportunity to develop pragmatic issues applied to Group Practices, Mental Health, Long-term Care, Hospitals, Ambulatory Care, and with this issue, Human and Social Services. The third year of *HMQ* will start off with specially applied issues to marketing for Health Maintenance Organizations and other forms of pre-paid health services. During the third year of publication the *Health Marketing Quarterly* will also publish a special issue of the Proceedings of the American College of Health Care Marketing Symposium '85. Our intent is to continually expand The Haworth Press marketing series to include the new *Journal of Professional Services Marketing, Psychotherapy Marketing & Practice Development Reports,* a text of *Readings and Cases in Health Care Marketing,* and the *Handbook of Health Care Advertising.* Information on all of these new marketing resources can be obtained directly from The Haworth Press, Inc.

INTRODUCTION TO THE HUMAN AND SOCIAL SERVICE MARKETING ISSUE

There is no sector of the health care industry which is in a greater state of change than human and social service agencies and programs. The emphasis on attempting to control the Federal Deficit has created economic policies related to containing, and in many cases, trimming social service budgets. The human and social service director is faced with a period of history when social consciousness and liberal thought has taken a back position to the desire for a strong economy and defense. Unfortunately, when we allocate monies and energies towards these goals there are significant opportunity costs in cutting social services. This has become very evident when we discuss such programs for such groups as the elderly, single parents, children, poor, handicapped, and minorities.

Many of the existing human and social services were expanded

xi

and reinforced during the Great Society periods of the 1960s and 1970s. In addition, these agencies became very dependent upon governmental funding. During the 1980s these programs have become the major target of cuts in funding and attempts at cost containment. A more competitive environment for social services has materialized. The problem lies in the fact that there is a strong need for new management skills in order to thrive in this competitive environment. One of these skill areas is marketing.

Marketing has to be integrated with other management specialties such as finance, economics, human resource, policy, and planning. Marketing allows the human service manager to (1) better understand the complexities of their marketplace; (2) identify the most promising avenues to pursue for the service; and (3) strategically position the organization in the marketplace to achieve its new goals and objectives. Human and social service organizations have had to adapt to the new environment and, in order to survive and prosper, become active rather than just reactive.

Most people think that marketing is just a way to attract new clients. This is very unfortunate when discussing using marketing for human and social services. The truth is that many social services are already oversaturated and possess long waiting lists. Therefore, marketing becomes a much wider and even more useful tool. Marketing allows the human and social service to improve its image in the community; expand the network of resources within the human service marketplace; attract newer bases of board members and volunteers; expand funding resources to newer public and private avenues; and improve the communication link between the agency and its clients, media, government agencies, private corporations and foundations, other human services, and the general public.

This issue of the *Health Marketing Quarterly* supplies some excellent resources on using marketing effectively. Most of the articles are based on case studies by experienced practitioners.

INTRODUCTION TO THE ARTICLES OF 'MARKETING FOR HUMAN AND SOCIAL SERVICE AGENCIES'

The Editorial this time supplies the reader with some points on developing one of the newest forms of marketing in health care—advertising. It is estimated that the majority of human service organizations will be using some form of advertising by 1990. Most managers in human services are not trained in marketing. Therefore, when trying to use advertising as a marketing strategy it is important to plan out your marketing program. Following some basic principles can be helpful in making a more effective ad for the service. The Guest Editorial has been supplied by Robert H. Christmas, Associate Administrator, Ambulatory Care Services, San Francisco General Hospital. Mr. Christmas brings over twenty years experience in serving the poor and disadvantaged in our society. He shares his thoughts on the serious problem of access to care for the medically indigent adult population during these times of changing health care economics.

PART I: GENERAL HEALTH CARE MARKETING AND STRATEGIC MARKETING PLANNING

The first article by Dr. Donald Dodson, Director of the Center for Management Development at the John A. Walker College of Business, supplies a thorough literary review of the development of health care marketing. Over 373 articles were reviewed for his research and they supported the continued embryonic stage of the development of health care marketing. The *Health Marketing Quarterly* is continuing the evolution into phase two of health care marketing—applications and tools for practitioners.

One of the first steps in marketing a human and social service organization is to develop a thorough strategic marketing plan. The second article by Dr. Vincent Faherty, Associate Professor in the School of Social Work at the University of Missouri-Columbia, provides a detailed outline of the major components of developing a social service marketing plan. A case example is applied to the Senior Care Corporation, Inc. in Middlevale, Missouri.

PART II: MARKETING RESEARCH AND TARGETING

As part of this marketing planning process a key element is the completion of a marketing audit. By conducting a systematic and periodic market audit, an organization remains current with the threats and opportunities posed by its marketplace, and can assess how these changes will affect their market position. The third article by

Dr. John Yankey, Professor at the School of Applied Social Sciences at Case Western Reserve University; Nancy Koury, Coordinator of Case Management Services at Breckenridge Village in Willoughby, Ohio; and Diana Young, Program Manager of the Impaired Driver Program at Alcoholism Services of Cleveland, Inc., in Cleveland, Ohio, provide a case study of developing a marketing audit. The audit is applied to the case study of Breckenridge Village, a non-profit retirement community in northeastern Ohio.

The new competitive environment is putting tremendous pressure on human service marketers to develop strategies which are segmentation-oriented. Marketing research supplied the framework for selecting a more concentrated targeting approach. The fourth article by Dr. Dennis McDermott, Associate Professor of Marketing at Virginia Commonwealth University in Richmond, Virginia, demonstrates a case study application of the use of marketing research. Via the use of focus groups and personal interviews research is compiled for an Adolescent Substance Abuse Program.

Another fine article by John Yankey, Diana Young, and Nancy Koury provides an illustration of how Alcoholism Services of Cleveland, Inc., a non-profit United Way member agency, utilized targeting and marketing research in the development of a consumer-focused promotional tool. A promotional brochure was developed through the use of marketing research information and select targeting in this fifth article in the journal.

PART III: MARKETING STRATEGIES—MARKETING MIX, POSITIONING AND SALESMANSHIP

One of the basic principles of marketing is the use of the marketing mix for developing marketing strategies. These components are typically called the five Ps of marketing. The five Ps include developing marketing strategies applied to select characteristics of PRODUCT, PLACE, PRICE, PROMOTION, and PEOPLE. As a special contribution to the *Health Marketing Quarterly,* the sixth article was developed by Ms. Rosanna Pribilovics, Associate Director, and in collaboration with Ira Okun, Executive Director, of the Family Service Agency of San Francisco. This fine sixth article describes how one of the oldest and most respected human service agencies in California utilized these five components of the marketing mix to continually enhance the agency's market position.

The seventh article is written by Gregory Nelson, Executive Director, and Mary Beth Barbaro of SERCO, a marketing and production firm in Dayton, Ohio, solely committed to mental health. A large proportion of human and social services are related to mental health. Over the years, the greatest obstacle to marketing mental health services has been the stigma associated with mental health services. This excellent article demonstrates a case study of how to position the organization for overcoming this stigma while promoting specific services. The case is applied to five participating mental health organizations located in Indiana, Illinois, Kentucky, Ohio, and Oklahoma.

The eighth article by Dr. Constantine G. Kledaras, Professor in the Department of Social Work and Correctional Services at East Carolina University, in Greenville, North Carolina, demonstrates a need for the social work profession to reflect upon their need for salesmanship. A knowledge of good salesmanship is lacking, according to Dr. Kledaras, in the repertoire of a social worker. An analysis of the advertising field is discussed in relation to good salesmanship being an ingredient to successful advertising. The author examines the premise that knowledge of advertising could enhance the profession of social work.

PART IV: SELECT RESEARCH CASES—HOSPICE CARE, PARENTING, AND DEINSTITUTIONALIZATION

One of the newest forms of human and social services has been the development of hospices. An advantage of using hospices has been marketed in relation to their cost-effectiveness based on the number of hospital days saved by using a hospice for terminally ill patients. The ninth article by Kathleen Oji-McNair, health consultant, and in association with Dr. Robert Goldman and Michael Tscheu, examines all costs of both traditional care and hospice care. The study indicates that the cost savings may not be as great as first surmised. However, the base of cost savings along with the hospices' value to the emotional and social aspects of the dying patient and their families presents a strong marketing strategy.

The tenth article by Jacques Bourgeois, President, Demand Research Consultants, Inc. and Barbara Helm, Education Consultant, Health Promotion Directorate, Health and Welfare Division of Canada, in Ottawa, Canada, examines parents' informational requirements on child rearing. Since one of the most important human service areas is related to parenting, basic findings regarding information sources medium, and types used by parents are presented. Marketing demands a good psychographic profile of the client base which is served in order to more effectively target and promote services. The findings of the study are further supplemented with differentiating characteristics such as language, community size, socio-economic status, and sexual distribution for parenting. The department of Health and Welfare in Canada has been doing some extensive research on identifying parents' perceptions of their information requirements with respect to child raising. These informational needs are closely tied to alcohol and drug issues. They can form the framework for a client profile and successful marketing plan for parenting and interrelated services.

The eleventh, and last article, in this issue is written by Dr. Salvatore Imbrogno, Professor, College of Social Work, The Ohio State University, Columbus, Ohio. One of the major new service areas for human and social service agencies is follow-care for those who have been institutionalized. A significant aspect of this problem is the availability of adequate living arrangements that promote individual growth and development, provide professional support and care, and elicit the concern of members in the community who will provide these living arrangements. The result of this study is that human service agencies involved in this service area can make decisions on placement based on knowledge, information, technology, and cost. Human service professionals can better serve their clients, and thus, raise the level of client satisfaction.

The journal provides some excellent case studies and methodologies for better understanding your clients' needs; planning the marketing activities; and developing marketing strategies. I hope the issue provides valuable information for better managing and marketing your human and social service.

William J. Winston
Editor

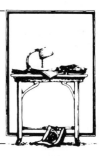

Key Points of Developing
an Advertisement for Human Services

During the last couple of years I have had the opportunity to be a speaker, panelist, paper presenter, and committee member at major meetings around the country. These activities have created a communication link with doctors, administrators, and practitioners in most major delivery areas of the health care industry. They have also provided me with the opportunity to see the explosive growth of interest in marketing around the country in all service sectors of the economy. The interest is intensifying during the second half of the 1980s. One of the most often asked questions I receive is about developing advertisements for select human services. In response to these inquiries, I have edited a new reference text for The Haworth Press on how to develop effective advertisements. Advertisements were collected from advertising agencies and health marketers from all over the country. It is interesting that effective advertising has begun to be used by almost every medical and health specialty. I estimate that over 500 million dollars per year will be spent by the health care industry on advertising by 1990. Since a large majority of health practitioners have never been trained in developing ads, I would like to share some basic principles for putting together an effective ad. A more complete description and multiple examples are provided in the new text.

PURPOSE OF ADVERTISING

The major purpose of advertising is to communicate an idea to a select target group. Advertising can only guide people's perceptions of a human service until they use it for the first time. It can really do only one thing: *It can convince a logical prospect for a human service to try it one time!* It cannot sell to someone who has no need for the service, satisfy a client, nor save a badly operated service.

The basic premise for every good ad is to "KEEP IT SIMPLE!" Unfortunately, this premise is so simple that most people perceive good advertising as having to be complex. Simple pictures, copy, and information can go a long way. For example, one of the most successful commercials on television was for the tourist trade in the Caribbean. The pictures showed a man strolling along a beautiful beach with just the sound of the waves in the background. At the end of the commercial, the words—Come See the Caribbean—appeared. It was simple in every way . . . and effective!

GOALS OF ADVERTISING

Advertising is directed to achieving the following:

a. Educating publics as to the need for a service;
b. Creating an awareness that the service exists;
c. Positioning the human service as unique among its competitors;
d. Creating referrals to the organization;
e. Stimulating select publics to try the service; and
f. Improving the financial viability of the organization and meeting the health needs of the community.

Advertising will not provide for a successful service. The delivery of the service must be provided effectively after advertising stimulates someone to try the service for the first time. The major success of any marketing campaign is the referral based upon client satisfaction.

TYPES OF ADVERTISING CHANNELS

Advertising can be initiated in different forms. Some of these advertising channels include: television, radio, newspapers, journals, direct mail, billboards, yellow pages, shopper/pennysavers, directories, transit space, posters, etc. The major criteria for which type of advertising channel is most appropriate depends on: the image the organization desires to promote, the target groups the service addresses, and any budget constraints. It is important to remember that advertising must be repeated in order to position the organization into the minds of the consumer. For example, many consumer behavior studies have proven that it takes a minimum of four to five repetitive ads for a consumer to try a service for the first time.

KEY STEPS IN WRITING AN ADVERTISEMENT

1. GET ATTENTION: Nobody is anxiously waiting to read or hear your advertisement. In addition, the advertising community is saturated. Your advertisement must get attention quickly by your target groups and have a lasting effect. This is especially important when most people will spend only about ten seconds reading print ad or fifteen seconds listening to an ad. Therefore, uniqueness through a headline, color scheme, graphical design, typeset, slogans, or pictures can be effectively portrayed.

2. DEMONSTRATE AN ADVANTAGE: The ad must answer the question, "What will this health service provide for me?" The consumer must be educated as to how the service will affect them physically or emotionally. Most of the time this is done through the copy of the ad. Copy must be kept short, but potent. The copy should explain to the potential clients about the benefit to be derived from trying the service.

3. PROVE AN ADVANTAGE: After the uniqueness of the services is demonstrated, some facts must be provided to validate these advantages. For example, if you claim your staff is of high quality, make sure their degrees or past positions are identified. Another ex-

ample would be to state that your fees are reasonable. Prove it by expressing the exact fees. A theme to remember would be to "always see the ad from the eyes of the consumer rather than from the perspective of the originator of the ad."

4. PERSUADE PEOPLE TO TAKE ADVANTAGE: After stating some form of factual information about proving the validity of why people should try the service, the ad must persuade the client to try it. Plan the ad to persuade the organization's toughest target group rather than the easiest ones. The persuasion aspect of the ad must bring the client to the point where they are aware, understand, and are ready to try it! An example would be to indicate that open enrollment will only occur during the month of November for your counseling service.

5. CALL FOR ACTION: Now that the consumer is almost ready to try the service, the ad should ask the consumer to take some form of action in contacting the service. For example, the ad can ask people to call a phone number, send in a coupon, come by and visit, or come to an open house. The idea is to have the consumer become aware of the service; realize the advantages of trying the service; and be stimulated to actually take an action and try the service for one time.

6. DO YOUR OWN ROUGH DRAFT OF THE AD: Take the time to try writing the ad with your team before using an advertising agency. Your team is the only one who truly understands the image or positioning advantages of the organization within the health community. Then take the copy to the ad agency for professional development and refinement.

7. TASKS OF AN AGENCY: There are thousands of advertising and public relations firms. The agency is mainly responsible for planning the advertising campaign with you; selecting and contracting for the type of media channel (i.e., television versus radio) which will produce the best results; prepare the advertising copy, layout, photography, and any artwork; produce the final ads for your approval; and takes care of all placement functions of the ad with, for example, the television or radio stations.

CONCLUSIONS

Creating a communications message which relates to the needs of your clients and placing the ad in the most effective media channel which serves these groups are the secrets to a good advertisement.

The ad must be represented in a manner which understands the behavior and values of your consumers. A good ad should include: information about the service; a clear statement which expresses the advantages of the service; and a creative and attention-getting presentation. These ingredients are based on two premises: *simplicity and believability.* Express an advertisement that has some substance but presented in a clear, concise, and simple fashion. Nothing should take away from the client remembering the name of the service and what you offer. Unfortunately, many ads get so carried away with sophisticated graphics and artwork that the main purpose of the ad is lost in the crowd!

These basic principles are the backbone to creating successful ads. They can be helpful as a simplistic guideline in developing an effective advertisement. After the client has tried your service for the first time, it is up to the quality of the service to assist in developing the important referral base and repeat usage patterns.

William J. Winston
Editor

GUEST EDITORIAL

Medically Indigent Adults: Access to Care?

Robert H. Christmas

The Federal Government, particularly for the thirty year period (1945-1975), developed health legislation that reflected in most instances, the main health and social concerns of society. A few examples:

Date	Concerns	Legislation
1946	Inadequate Health Facilities	PL79-725 Hill Burton
1963	Adequate Manpower	PL 88-129 Professional School Construction
1965	Access to Health Services	Title XVIII & XIX Social Security Amendments
1973	Cost Containment	PL93-222 HMO's
1974	Planning/Resource Allocation	PL93-641 HSA's

The government's legislative response to the "access" issues precipitated, in my opinion, a provider/consumer reaction that well may change the health care industry for many years.

Title XVII and XIX, provided a mechanism to make accessible

Robert H. Christmas is Associate Administrator of Ambulatory Care Services, San Francisco General Hospital, San Francisco, CA.

7

health care services to specific groups historically excluded from the "main stream" of health care. These groups, the poor and the aged, were afforded the opportunity, within certain parameters, to select the health care "plan of their choice" realizing inability to pay for health services was ostensibly, no longer a barrier in seeking quality health care services.

The government's and consumer response to the access issue has contributed, in part, to the dilemma we are currently experiencing in the health care industry. The dilemma is that most advances made were achieved at high cost—among the highest in the world—and low efficiency. Society's concern with cost is ever apparent within the past 6-8 years, particularly the cost of health care services. We should expect, as is the case, public policy reflecting these concerns. Public policy, in any form, can be defined as a means of ordering priorities within established constraints. In light of the above, we have witnessed various attempts by government (Local, State, and Federal) to contain and where possible, curtail health resources, particularly those resources earmarked for the poor. (The Reagan Administration's New Federalism strategy, which assumes that State and Local government will finance Federal funding cuts in health care services, is drawing wide skepticism.)

This competitive strategy for controlling health care costs can't be anything but threatening to the institutions experiencing a disproportionate share of the cost of care for the medically indigent patient.

The emerging reality here is that the competitive strategy is really a mad scramble for a larger share of the private market and has only limited relevance to the cause of cost control.

That piece of competitive doctrine that puts the consumer of care at risk just isn't real when applied to poor people. You can't reasonably impose significant financial risk on people who cannot afford to finance their care in the first place. Therefore the "risk" experienced by the poor is to be mandated to receive care at institutions where they find themselves financially acceptable.

We, of course, know that the only institutions that fund this group, the medically indigent, "financially acceptable," are those institutions (usually city/county hospitals) legally bound to do so.

Stricter eligibility standards, regarding participating in programs, maximum payment allowances to providers and overall services reductions have further narrowed the options this targeted group can exercise. This narrowing of options has resulted in an emerging "two-tiered" system of health care.

What is meant by "two-tiered" health care? If it means fish sticks instead of lobster, and ward accommodation instead of private, that is one thing. If it means making it difficult for the "second tier" types to get inside our hospitals, that is another thing. If it means consigning all of the country's indigent to understaffed and underequipped public hospitals, that is something else again.

The dilemma comes into focus immediately when it is related to specific situations. Does that mean that we shouldn't give a liver transplant to the father of a young family when the father doesn't have a job? Does it mean a premature infant of an AFDC mother can't get admitted to a neonatal intensive care unit? Does this mean we should take dialysis away from the elderly?

Moving overtly to two-tiers poses significant ethical as well as political problems. Many private practitioners finesse the ethical issue by limiting their practices using socio-economic criteria. *The disenfranchised patient becomes somebody else's problem!* Acceptance of the idea of a two-tiered system of care seems to be gaining ground in our country, but only among those who feel they will land safely on the first tier.

The quality of patient care, particularly care directed toward the poor, has always been in conflict with the government's ever increasing emphasis on cost control.

Apparently, the health care problems of the poor need to worsen before they are addressed nationally, and from all indication, the problems will worsen!

I am sure we all agree that the problem of health care *in*accessibility is national in scope, everybody is affected. Whatever our roles in the health care system, we all believe deeply that our society must not let its poor suffer or die for want of much needed health care services.

What is needed for long term stability is a plan for sharing the cost of indigent care among all the parties at interest—government at all levels, business and industry, providers of services, consumers of service, insurers and taxpayers—so that all are paying their fair share.

Unless we can develop mechanisms to provide quality health care services to this growing segment of the population, circumstances will, most probably, precipitate the type of solution nobody wants.

PART I: GENERAL HEALTH CARE MARKETING AND STRATEGIC MARKETING PLANNING

Health care marketing has entered its second phase of development. During the first five years we spent most of our time explaining what marketing is and why it is important to use for human services. During the last two years we have begun to see marketing expand into the second phase of developing, training, and utilizing marketing resources. Marketers are being trained for the health care industry. New marketing methodologies are being created. Some sophisticated marketing techniques are beginning to be utilized throughout the industry. The third phase is quite a way off yet. This forthcoming phase of development will see plenty of experienced health marketers who have advanced to the stages of sophistication whereby strategy development, financial analysis, and computer utilization are interwoven. There is a strong correlation between the evolution of health marketing and Alvin Toffler's three waves of industrial development. It is important for human and social service managers to be aware of the historical and current status of marketing in their industry. The first article reviews the literary status through 1983. It is a pleasure to know that the *Health Marketing Quarterly* has emerged during the two years to bridge the gaps indicated in this literary search.

The most important aspect of developing a marketing program for human and social service programs is to write a formal marketing plan. A marketing plan outlines a formal plan of marketing action for the human service program. It also brings our marketing resources into perspective and organization. The second article in this section supplies the basic ingredients for developing such a plan.

WJW

Health Care Marketing: Advancements But No Cigar

Don C. Dodson, PhD

INTRODUCTION

During the past decade health care marketing has received considerable attention in health administration literature. Because it is still in an embryonic stage, the levels of sophistication in health care marketing research vary significantly from one functional area of health administration to another. However, it is generally recognized that hospitals are further advanced in health care marketing thought, research and implementation than any other health discipline within the health delivery system. (For additional information, see Steven W. Brown, "Candid Observations on the Status of Health Services Marketing," *Journal of Health Care Marketing,* Vol. 3, No. 3 (Summer 1983), pp. 45-52.)

Today, many hospitals employ full-time marketing directors at the department head or vice-presidential levels; the American Marketing Association has a special section devoted exclusively to health care marketing; and there are at least two journals devoted exclusively to health care marketing. Nationally, there has been a proliferation of health care marketing training programs, seminars, newsletters, consulting activities and books produced on the subject. Nevertheless, no systematic study has been undertaken to evaluate published research in this new discipline and to determine its methodology, usefulness or practical utility. This study is an attempt to fill that void.

This study utilized two established computer searches, Dialog and Medline. The Dialog searches both the Health Planning and Admin-

---

Don C. Dodson is currently Professor of Health Care Management and Director of the Center for Management Development at the John A. Walker College of Business, Appalachian State University, Boone, NC. He has been Executive Director of the American Academy of Health Administration and was the founding editor of *The Journal of Health Care Marketing.*

© 1985 by The Haworth Press, Inc. All rights reserved.   *13*

istration Database from business and health journals. Medline is produced by the U.S. National Library of Medicine and is the most popular database for health administration in use today. It was felt that the combination of these two searches should reveal all major published research in health care marketing. From these initial searches, a review of the literature printouts was conducted and an analysis of each appropriate article was conducted.

RESEARCH

For the purposes of this study, the following criteria were used to determine what research is.

1. Studies and research have been broadly defined as those sets of activities which provide systematically assembled information concerning health care marketing, its components and environment.
2. A set of activities was considered research when the following ingredients were, for the most part, present:
    2.1. There existed a statement of the area of investigation or problem, present or implicit.
    A statement of goals or objectives existed, present or implicit.
    A statement of assumptions existed, present or implicit.
    2.2. Data or information was systematically collected and presented.
    2.3. Analysis of the date or information was attempted and presented.
    2.4. Findings and conclusions were presented.
    2.5. There was a potential for generalization upon the experience.

RESOURCES

Even though health care marketing is a rapidly emerging discipline in the field of health administration, no systematic review of the literature or research can be identified. The only general resources that can be identified are *Health Care Marketing: An Annotated Bibliography,* published by the U.S. Department of Health,

Education and Welfare, Center for Disease Control, Bureau of Health Education, Atlanta, Georgia, March 1980 and *Health Marketing Resources* (updated). *Health Care Marketing: An Annotated Bibliography* consists of two-hundred fifty-six (256) entries, less than half of the published literature which exists today, and is generally descriptive. Moreover, it does not contain the latest or most significant materials available. *Health Marketing References* is more up-to-date, although a review indicates that some published research is not included. Nevertheless, it remains the best single bibliographic source that can be identified.

Therefore, this study is necessary to fill a void in the literature of a major emerging subfield of health care administration.

HOSPITAL MARKETING—AN OVERVIEW

In order to fully understand the current role and status of marketing in hospitals, it is important to briefly trace the development of hospital administration. Managerial theory and practice trace their roots to the Sumerians, the developers of a written language. Significant contributions have been made toward this development by individual organizations and nations, especially the Roman Catholic Church with its record-keeping; Diocletian's reorganization of the Roman Empire; and the development of the factory system. Modern management thought can be traced to scientific management and Max Weber's theories on bureaucracy.

Hospital administration, at least from an academic perspective, is traced to the first hospital administration program (graduate) at the University of Chicago in 1934. Prior to that time the common belief and practice was that hospitals and health institutions could be managed only by physicians. Some of that thought and practice still remain, especially in public health, but in hospitals it is now generally recognized that special training in management is a prerequisite for hospital administration. Today, over one-hundred (100) graduate hospital administration programs exist in the United States alone. Several colleges of business also offer health administration "tracks" within Master of Business Administration programs. According to the Association of University Programs in Health Administration, no degree program in health care marketing can be identified (*Annual Report,* Association of University Programs in Health Administration, Washington, DC, 1983).

Even though hospital administration is almost half a century old, it has still been slow to adopt and adapt business management specialties into the study of hospital administration. The curriculum in most university programs is based upon general management, with specific courses in finance or personnel (Don C. Dodson, "Graduate Hospital Program—A Review," Unpublished Report, College of Arts & Sciences, Auburn University, 1974). Therefore, it is not surprising that business management subfields have been slow to make their way into hospital management thought. By the mid-1970's, however, most subfields, such as personnel administration, information systems, office management, finance, etc., had become functional departments of most hospitals. When these departments are at a vice-presidential level in a hospital, they are usually filled by management generalists, not by trained specialists.

Marketing is the last of the subfield to be accepted as a functional discipline and the reasons for this are more complex than for the other subfields. There appear to be four major reasons why marketing has not historically been accepted by hospital administrators:

1. Lack of a perceived need.
2. Belief that marketing had no role in service organizations.
3. Misconceptions about the value of marketing.
4. The image of marketing. (See Richard M. Hodgetts and Dorothy M. Cascion, *Modern Health Care Administration,* New York: Academic Press, 1983, p. 440; and Don C. Dodson and B. J. Dunlap, "Public Health Marketing: Old Myths and New Realities," presented at the 1980 Annual Meeting of the American Public Health Association, New York.)

Marketing did not begin to gain acceptance into the health field until Philip Kotler introduced the concept of social marketing to the non-profit and health fields. Probably the most significant work in bringing the marketing concept to the academic disciplines of health administration was Kotler's *Marketing for Non Profit Organizations.* In this work, Kotler carefully brought the reader from the basics of marketing to case studies, beginning with the concept of marketing. His definition of marketing is still the basis for most definitions of health marketing:

Marketing is the analysis, planning, implementation, and con-

trol of carefully formulated programs designed to bring about
voluntary exchanges of values with target markets for the purpose of achieving organizational objectives.

It relies heavily on
designing the organization's offering in terms of the target
markets' needs and desires, and on using effective pricing,
communication and distribution to inform, motivate, and service the markets. (Philip Kotler, *Marketing for Non Profit
Organizations*, Englewood Cliffs, NJ: Prentice-Hall, 1975,
p. 5).

Kotler is now generally referred to in the literature as the ''Father of
Social Marketing.'' Because of Kotler's works others began to write
in this field..A typical example is *Marketing in Non Profit Organizations*, edited by Patrick J. Montana (New York: Amacom, 1978).

In his early works, Kotler emphasized that marketing should
broaden its scope. As early as 1969, in an article in the *Journal of
Marketing*, ''Broadening the Concept of Marketing,'' Kotler used
this theme. He wrote: ''When we come to the marketing function, it
is also clear that every organization performs marketing-like activities whether or not they are recognized as such.'' His arguments
were persuasive and many practitioners in the health field, especially hospital administrators, began reading Kotler's works.

The impact of the work of Philip Kotler in the late 1960's and
throughout the 1970's cannot be overstated in terms of where we are
in health care marketing today. His work is conceptual rather than
research-oriented, although it is clear that a research foundation was
present. The logic of his arguments and clear writing style led others
to apply his social marketing and ''broadening (of) the marketing
concept'' to health administration.

The first significant work in health care marketing was *Health
Care Marketing* by Robin MacStravic (USA: Aspen, 1975). By any
standard the book is not sophisticated and actually has little utility as
a practical or academic work. In fact, it is little more than a com-
pilation of other works. But the book does have significance when
viewed from an historical perspective. While it does not explain ex-
actly what marketing can do for a health organization, it does make
the point that there is value in marketing for these organizations.
Since the book was marketed by an aggressive publisher, it received
considerable attention from hospital administrators. This has directly led to a proliferation of hospital marketing seminars conducted by

Aspen Publishers and other organizations throughout the U.S. These seminars, although most cover only the basics of marketing, have been extremely successful in attracting large audiences.

Since late 1980, three journals devoted to health care marketing have been introduced. In late 1980's, the first, the *Journal of Health Care Marketing (JHCM)*, appeared. Almost immediately Aspen published another journal, The *Journal of Planning and Marketing*, although the main emphasis was on planning and the journal was on the market for less than a year. The other journal *Health Marketing Quarterly*, was only begun recently.

It should be noted that Wentworth Publishing's, *Profiles in Hospital Marketing*, has been successful, and although it advertises as a journal, it is a source only for advertising and promotional ideas. Thus, materials from *Profiles* will not be reviewed in this paper.

Several books have been published in the 1980's about health and hospital marketing, almost exclusively for practitioners. One of the most popular has been *Health Care Marketing, Issues and Trends*, (Philip D. Cooper, Ed., USA: Aspen, 1979). The book is a grouping of reprints that begins with articles dealing with the foundations of marketing, e.g., Section I is "The Emergence of Health Care Marketing" and the first article (by Cooper) is "What is Health Care Marketing?" This book is still widely used in hospitals, which reflects the continued usefulness of basic articles in health organizations.

Most of the books being published in health and hospital marketing are of the "how to" variety. A typical example is Norman H. McMillan's, *Marketing Your Hospital: A Strategy for Survival* (Chicago: American Hospital Association, no date). Again, the book begins by defining marketing, which is immediately followed by a heading, "Marketing Is Not A Four-Letter Word." Rubright and MacDonald's *Marketing Health and Human Services* (Aspen, 1981) provides down to earth examples and information and Hillestad and Berkowitz, *Health Care Marketing Plans: From Strategy to Action*, meets a new demand of combining marketing and strategic planning.

There are still relatively few books available in health care marketing, although this is one of the "hottest" areas in health administration today. This is partly attributable to the lack of expertise available for writing books and to the failure to understand and implement marketing on a sophisticated basis. Clearly, books in the field of health care and hospital marketing reveal the embryonic stage of development of the discipline.

Although books are useful tools to determine the level of sophistication of research in a discipline, articles, at least in this case, are a better determinant.

HOSPITAL MARKETING MATRIX

A matrix was developed to determine the relative number of articles in various health organizations and the specific marketing function which these articles addressed. A total of 373 articles were reviewed. The articles were selected from those listed in a Dialog search from the Health Planning and Administration Database. Several articles listed were not of the proper subject area and were not listed in the matrix.

The original matrix listed all marketing functions and all health organizations covered by the article. When articles discussed more than one function or organization, the dominant theme was listed. No article carried dual listing.

After an initial review and completion of the first matrix, several categories, in which only one or two total articles were found, were collapsed into a miscellaneous category. It should be noted that the category, "Generic," refers to either marketing or health institutions in their broadest sense and not to a particular function or organization. The "Miscellaneous" category includes articles about specific functions or organization but with too few references for a category listing on the matrix. The final matrix appears in Table 1.

The matrix did not reveal anything new to those familiar to the field, but should be important to students and to new practitioners. The matrix does, however, reinforce quantitatively what is the generally held view in the discipline; namely, that hospitals are the leading health institutions utilizing health care marketing and that health care marketing still reflects a rudimentary stage as it focuses on promotion, often to the exclusion of other aspects of the marketing mix.

One value in having the figures available in a modified matrix is that it brings into mental focus conclusions that may be difficult to reach *via* more abstract thinking processes. As an example, it is interesting to note that health care institutions that are operated on a more business-like basis, or ones that may indeed be for-profit organizations, reflect marketing literature more than do public sector

Table 1. A Matrix of Marketing Functions and Institutions from Selected Marketing Articles*

	Hospitals	Public Health	Medical Practice/Group Practice	Medical Records	Dental	Mental Health	Misc.	Generic	Total
Promotion	86	2	6	3	15	2	42	14	170
Product (Service)	2						1	1	4
Place (Location)	1								1
Price (Budget; Finance)	7						3		10
Interview	9		1				1	3	14
Editorial	4	1					1	3	9
Marketing Audit	10							2	12
General	15		6	1	5	2	4	8	41
Planning	11				1		6	2	20
Marketing Management (Organization)	11			2			1	2	16
Marketing Mix	3							1	4
Miscellaneous	35		3	1	6		20	7	72
Total	194	3	16	7	27	4	79	43	373

*Empty cells = 0

Note: The horizontal listing is for health institutions. The vertical listing is for marketing functions.

health institutions. For example, only three articles (one an editorial) were listed for public health, while 194 were listed for hospitals. This is somewhat ironic, too, because historically public health has been in the forefront of promoting (in the marketing sense) the concept of prevention before care, through the discipline and practice of health education. Public health also receives considerable free publicity through public service announcements, through programs to make its services known, and is actually funded by various levels of government to promote services.

Even though promotion articles dominate all categories, regardless of the type of institution, it is important to also note that more sophisticated marketing tools and strategies are employed by hospitals when compared to other health institutions. Articles on marketing audits, for example, appeared ten times in hospital literature but only twice in the literature of all other health organizations combined. Other examples in the matrix, such as marketing management and health planning and finance support the contention that not only are hospitals further developed in the quantity of literature published in health care marketing, but that the literature is more sophisticated.

Some of the imbalance in the figures presented in the matrix for hospital promotions is attributable to articles published by *Profiles in Hospital Marketing.* While these are indexed as articles, they are actually advertising and promotional ideas that are shared through the magazine by hospitals. Nevertheless, when these are factored out, the final totals are still heavily weighted in favor of hospital promotion articles.

The subject of health planning is another irony that the matrix brings into focus. Planning has long been held as a cornerstone of social and governmental services. This is especially true in health service administration since the 1966 Comprehensive Health Planning Act and later in 1974 with the creation of Health Systems Agencies. Apparently the connection between planning and marketing has not reached policy-making levels within public health.

Part of this can be explained by the education that health administrators receive. As noted by Clarke (Roberta N. Clarke, ''Marketing Health Care: Problems in Implementation,'' *Health Care Management Review,* Winter, 1978, p. 22), the most accepted courses of study for health administrators, the Master of Public Health (MPH), the Master of Health Administration (MHA), and the Master of Public Administration (MPA), do not generally require marketing courses. Clarke also notes that managerial positions are often filled or significantly influenced by physicians "when formal training not only lacks a marketing component, but often includes a chastisement of those availing themselves of the promotional benefits of marketing" (Clarke, p. 22). Public health has a greater number of physicians in managerial positions, often a legal requirement, than do other health institutions, especially hospitals. As the Master of Business Administration (MBA) continues to become a favored degree, both in hospitals and in group and dental practice management, it can be expected that administrators with academic backgrounds in marketing will be more willing to accept this new discipline than those without a familiarity with it.

The acceptance of marketing by hospital administrators over other health administrators is also reflected in the subscription figures of the *Journal of Health Care Marketing (JHCM)* the first journal devoted exclusively to health care marketing. Over 80 percent of the subscribers represent hospitals with less than 20 percent representing the public sector (Source: Bureau of Economic and Business Research, John A. Walker College of Business, Appalachian State University).

ARTICLES AND SUBJECTS—AN OVERVIEW

As might be expected after reviewing books in health care marketing, most articles do not reflect research findings or data sources. Some articles may indeed be based on research, but this is difficult to ascertain by reading them. The primary reason is probably due to the lack of research, but it is also due to the types of journals that accept health marketing articles. For example, the leading journal published by the American Hospital Association, *Hospitals,* has editorial policies which make it almost impossible to publish research articles. Often the health administration literature is more like a trade magazine. Research is often reserved for the clinically-oriented and scientific journals. This is a severe weakness in health administration literature.

A notable exception to the research rule is the *Journal of Health Care Marketing.* Most of the articles published in *JHCM* are research-based and all are refereed. However, the *JHCM* is not devoted exclusively to hospitals, so the total number of research articles about hospital marketing is limited.

Most of the articles reviewed still focus on: what marketing is; appeals for implementing marketing in hospitals; the value of marketing; or ideas or thoughts about marketing. Even articles on marketing audits are based on known information and no research about the use of audits is reflected in the published works, even though this does seem to be a topic of interest to hospital administrators.

SUMMARY AND CONCLUSIONS

That only a few articles on hospital marketing can be classified as research points out that health marketing is still generally a discipline that has a long way to go before it reaches the professional levels found in other hospital administration subfields. It is reasonable to assume, too, that health marketing is here to stay, that it will grow and that more research will be forthcoming. But it is also reasonable to assume that until university programs begin to graduate health care marketers the field will be severely limited in its ability to conduct market research.

The literature clearly reflects a field that is neither sophisticated nor research-oriented. Most of the literature is still "down and dirty," is generally descriptive, and is based on personal observation or opinion. It is likely that since university programs in health administration are not meeting the manpower needs in health marketing, it will be a long time before health marketing is fully understood by health practitioners.

BIBLIOGRAPHY

Annual Report. Association of University Professors in Health Administration, Washington, D. C.: 1983.
Cooper, Philip D., Ed. *Health Care Marketing.* USA: Aspen, 1979.
Dodson, Don C., "Graduate Hospital Programs—A Review," Auburn, Ala.: Auburn University, College of Arts & Sciences, 1974.
_____ and B. J. Dunlap, "Public Health Marketing: Old Myths and New Realities," N. Y.: Annual Meeting of the American Public Health Association, 1980.
Hodgetts, Richard M.; Cascion, Dorothy M. *Modern Health Care Administration.* New York: Academic Press, 1983.
Kotler, Philip A. *Marketing for Non Profit Organizations.* Englewood Cliffs, N. J.: Prentice-Hall, 1975.
McMilian, Norman H. *Marketing Your Hospital: A Strategy for Survival.* Chicago: American Hospital Association, n.d.
MacStravic, Robin. *Health Care Marketing.* USA: Aspen, 1975.
Montana, Patrick J., Ed. *Marketing in Non Profit Organization.* New York: Amacom, 1978.

First Steps First: Developing a Marketing Plan Case Example: Senior Care Corporation, Inc.

Vincent Edward Faherty, DSW, MBA

It is an understatement to note that many social service administrators are in a dilemma these days. They are quite aware that *competition* is the latest and potentially most serious threat that is assailing them—competition from public, non-profit and proprietary social service agencies. In the face of this threat, these same administrators appear quite uncomfortable with the clear and consistent advice they receive from colleagues, from professional associations and from the popular press. This advice can be summarized as: "Market yourself creatively but aggressively . . . advertise your services in the media!" "But," these administrators' respond, "we are professionals helping people, not salesmen selling sausages!"

The threats and emotions may be painfully real, but the dilemma is false . . . for two reasons. First, a marketing approach to social services delivery is unequivocally professional. Kotler defines marketing as that ". . . human activity directed at satisfying needs and wants through the exchange process."[1] Whether that exchange process is oriented towards profit or non-profit goals is irrelevant. What is relevant, however, is the marketing perspective of satisfying consumer needs/wants through some product or service—which is supposed to be the ultimate goal of any social welfare agency established to promote societal well-being. The second reason why the administrators' dilemma is false is the fact that marketing should *not* be equated with advertising in the public media. This is a very common misunderstanding which can easily result in costly and misdi-

Vincent Edward Faherty, Associate Professor, School of Social Work, University of Missouri, Columbia, MO.

rected attempts to "market" an agency in the public environment.

The social service administrator who wants to deliver effective services—comprehensive in nature and relevant to identified needs—in the most cost efficient manner should have what every good business executive has: an updated marketing plan. This article will attempt to provide an outline of what such a marketing plan should contain for the social service agency in the case example which follows.

A CASE EXAMPLE:
THE SENIOR CARE CORPORATION, INC.[2]

The Senior Care Corporation, Inc. (SCC) is a not-for-profit social service agency initiated and legally incorporated by a group of twelve community residents of Middlevale, Missouri. This group of twelve have been constituted as the corporate Board of Directors of SCC and they are fairly representative of most community-based boards, i.e., their ranks include a banker, lawyer, clergyman, social worker, physician, nurse, several business executives, two homemakers, and a graduate student from a local university. The primary goal of SCC is to provide total residential care to a specialized client group: the mentally retarded/developmentally disabled (MR/DD) senior citizen. The entire Board of Directors is personally involved in this unique target group of clients because each one either has a family member who is both aged and MR/DD, or is a professional working in that area of social service practice.

Approximately eighteen months previous to this time, the present Board of Directors had coalesced together because of a serious community incident which resulted in the death of a seventy five year old mentally retarded woman who had slipped through the "safety net" of the social welfare system. By means of an extensive community campaign for the past twelve months, the Board has been able to raise one hundred thousand dollars in donations and has a commitment for an additional three hundred thousand dollars from a local bank in conjunction with the Small Business Administration. The bank will offer a twenty year note at fifteen percent annual interest.

At this point in time, six months after legal incorporation, construction is almost complete on a twenty-four bed residential facility located on a large, wooded plot of land two miles outside the city of Middlevale. If all continues according to plan the facility will be licensed by the Missouri Division of Aging and will be certified as an "intensive care facility" eligible for funding under the Medicaid program. A tentative, non-contractual agreement with the state agency will assure, to a relative degree of certainty, that clients will be referred whenever an opening exists. SCC will receive a per diem cost of care rate of ninety-seven dollars per resident.

During the previous week, the Board of Directors hired an experienced executive director who will be assuming total operational responsibility for the program within the next thirty days. This new executive director raised several important issues during his interview, one in particular referred to the pro forma budget for the facility. As projected by the finance subcommittee of the Board, the income statement for SCC after one full year of operation showed four thousand dollars in excess revenue after accounting for all operating expenses and the interest on the bank note. This four thousand dollars would constitute the beginning of a reserve fund to be utilized for future program developments.

The executive director noted to the Board that the positive cash flow and the resultant reserve fund was based on several assumptions:

1. the facility will be able to maintain a resident population at a minimum of ninety percent of capacity depending solely on referrals from the Missouri Division of Aging;
2. the State will not lower its per diem cost of care rate because of some public budget crisis;
3. a need for this program exists now and will continue to exist in the near and mid-term future; and, finally,
4. if there is competition in the immediate community for the consumers of this service, the need for the service is greater than/equal to the amount of service available.

Upon further discussion, the Board decided to develop a marketing plan. This decision, unique for a social service agency, came about because of the concerns expressed by the new executive director and because of the persuasive arguments of the small group of business people on the Board.

What follows is not the marketing plan itself—which would be too lengthy and too case-specific to offer much applicability to other contexts—but, rather, an outline of the major components that make up a marketing plan and a summary of the essential questions to be asked/answered in each section.[3]

DEVELOPING A MARKETING PLAN

Step One: Situation Analysis

One of the classic articles in marketing by Levitt challenges the corporate chief executive officer or the social service administrator to answer clearly the question: what business are you in?[4] This is not simply a semantic clarification. The question and answer are of critical strategic importance. Levitt's point, transposed to a social service context, is that specific social service program offerings can be transient while the basic market needs (i.e., client needs) are enduring. Thus ". . . a horse carriage company will go out of business as soon as the automobile is invented. But the same company, defined as a people moving business, would switch from horse carriage manufacturer to car manufacturer."[5] In our case example, an important clarification would seem to be that SCC is in the business of providing residential care for special-needs clients. This, then, would allow SCC to adjust its programming, e.g., to provide temporary, "respite" care for the aged MR/DD client rather than long term care; or to serve MR/DD clients who are younger than sixty-five years of age; or to re-define totally what "special needs" it wishes to relate to in light of changing demographic or financial factors. This is the "marketing approach" in its purest form: to be able to adjust to varying client/consumer needs.

Once this question has been answered clearly and substantively, this first step in the development of a marketing plan then requires the explication of the present state of the agency including history, organizational structure, immediate community environment, strengths and weaknesses of the agency itself and its programs, and, finally, the threats and opportunities present in the external environment. In the case example, the fact that SCC is a new, untested agency would be a critical factor to consider here. Other factors of equal importance would be: the risk involved in total dependence on a single source of client referral; how extensive is the nursing home network in the community since this sub-system provides a potential (or real) competitive threat; and, finally, how many actual clients, including their financial capability, exist now and five years from now in the community.

Obviously, this first step in the marketing plan demands a significant amount of objective market research—the kind that, in most cases, should be purchased on contract from a university or private marketing research group.

Step Two: Marketing Objectives

At this second stage in the market plan, the task is to decide in what direction the agency should proceed. In the private sector, the corporate business executive must choose between (or at least rank order) three distinct directions: increase sales volume, seize greater market shares or gain maximum profit per sale. The social agency executive has the same set of choices although the language may be different: will the agency strive to provide as much service as possible to the largest number of people who need the service? or will the agency become the identified ''expert'' on providing a particular service and thus ''dominate'' the community by being the ''best''? or, will the agency stay small in a planned manner and gain maximum exposure by focusing only on a limited number of carefully selected clients.

It is true that these three choices are not totally exclusive of each other, and, further, that the nature of the service provided may dictate one particular direction over another. The point, however, is still germane: a general marketing goal must be chosen consciously (or at least a set of goals rank-ordered) and this goal direction will influence a highly-specific set of behaviorally-stated marketing objectives. In our case example, the Board needs to make some hard decisions about whether or not they will accept private clients referred by their own families rather than by the state authorities; whether they envision any expansion five or ten years from now with two or three additional centers operational; or, whether they perceive themselves as a specialized ''laboratory'' providing innovative, ''state of the art'' programming to a carefully selected client population. These questions in no way exhaust the total range of directional goals that are possible for SCC, but they should demonstrate the kind of exploration that must occur in order to provide a set of concise, observable and meaningful objectives.

Step Three: Marketing Strategies

In this section of plan, the task is to project a comprehensive and coordinated strategy that will achieve the identified objectives and goals. This step is a critical one and there are, literally, volumes written on this one step alone.[6] Thus, this article can present only the barest elements of some fundamental issues that need to be addressed in choosing marketing strategies. The reader is advised to explore the wide spectrum of available literature for more in-depth information. For the purposes of this summary-type article, however, three points need to be emphasized.

1. Alternative marketing strategies. Based on the premise that one objective can give rise to several means/strategies to achieve it successfully, it becomes apparent that energy must be expended in the listing of all possible strategies before the decision is made on which one or two are feasible. This is a time-consuming process requiring the creative efforts usually of a group of knowledgeable staff.

2. Segmentation, Targeting, Positioning. These concepts, which are found in every business marketing text, must be understood and adapted to the social service agency because of their utility in strategy selection. *Segmentation* relates to the need to subdivide the potential client market into distinct and meaningful subsets of clients on the assumption that these subsets might demand separate marketing activities in order to reach them (e.g., segments of potential clients who live in urban, suburban and rural areas). *Targeting* involves the agency's decision to select and concentrate on one or more of the market segments in the effort to serve them most effectively and efficiently (e.g., targeting in on only the urban clients to the exclusion of rural and suburban). *Positioning* can be explained in the context of how the agency views itself vis-à-vis other, similar agencies in the community or region. Thus, an agency attempts to be positioned as either the "leader" in terms of staff size, number of clients served, etc.; the "challenger" to the leader; the "follower" who observes and learns from the leader and challenger; or, finally, the "nicher" who is content to specialize narrowly on one sub-area and be very good at what it does.

3. Product, Price, Promotion, Place. This component is concerned with the so-called "marketing mix"—the completed product or service that is offered in its entirety to the consumer for sale. The marketing mix can be most easily understood when one buys a box of "Wheaties" in a supermarket. The consumer buys Wheaties rather than a box of "Rice Krispies" at a competitive sale price, probably due to a newspaper advertisement, and the purchase takes place at a supermarket. That sale was completed because of an inter-related set of marketing decisions made many months before on the issues of product/price/promotion/place. All of these elements of strategic marketing might not appear equally important for the services provided by a social agency but all do demand some attention. Promotion is certainly vital, and at this stage in the market plan development the contracted services of an advertising agency should be utilized.

Step Four: Implementation

As any administrator can testify, whether in the public, non-profit or private sectors no plan can be *operationalized* without the commitment of people, time and resources. Thus, a marketing plan for a social service agency, if it is to be considered seriously, must provide for the allocation of staff to collect and interpret available information; a realistic time frame to realize accomplishments; and financial resources to pay for contracted services, materials and products. The fact that a marketing plan is a *plan* needing to be operationalized (*not* some vague philosophical principle expressed by the Board) is a point that can be overlooked easily by a social service agency executive not used to working with such a document.

Step Five: Evaluation

Unless imposed from above or from some external authority, one's own peculiar style of administrative leadership will probably dictate the type of control mechanism utilized to gauge the effectiveness of a marketing plan. A common technique in business is some from a PERT chart which assigns and monitors responsibilities and targets within the time frame of weeks, months, or quarters. A quantitative rather than a qualitative approach is considered more useful because of the very nature of the marketing plan. Again, the pure quantitative measures may cause some discomfort in social service administrators, who are used to more qualitative factors. The market plan itself, however, must be seen for what it is and what it is not: it is a means to be more responsive to client needs and this should be measurable in numerical terms . . . it is not a substitute for the agency's general goal statement which, due to the nature of human need, must be more humanistic and qualitative in structure.

CONCLUSION

Jay Conrad Levinson, in his excellent and provocative book entitled, *Guerilla Marketing,* advises that the three most important marketing secrets can be summarized in three words: commitment, investment and consistent. The real danger point he cautions, is when the well-conceived marketing plan begins to generate results for the tendency then is to abandon the plan, ease up on the commitment to a marketing approach, reallocate resources to other parts of the organization and lose the consistency of the promotional messages before the community. To avoid that situation, Levinson would have every administrator tack up on the wall someplace his "ten truths you must never forget:"[7]

1. The market is constantly changing
2. People forget fast
3. Your competition isn't quitting
4. Marketing strengthens your identity
5. Marketing is essential to survival and growth
6. Marketing enables you to hold on to your old customers
7. Marketing maintains morale
8. Marketing gives you an advantage over competitors who have ceased marketing
9. Marketing allows your business to continue operating
10. You have invested money that you stand to lose.

NOTES AND REFERENCES

1. Philip Kotler, *Marketing Management* (Fourth Edition, Englewood Cliffs, New Jersey: Prentice-Hall International, 1980), p. 19.

2. The Senior Care Corporation is a composite picture of several social service agencies.

3. There is no "ideal" or universally accepted marketing plan outline. For other approaches see: Jay Diamond and Gerald Pintel, *Principles of Marketing* (Englewood Cliffs, New Jersey: Prentice Hall, 1972; Herman Holtz, *The Secrets of Practical Marketing for Small Business* (Englewood Cliffs, New Jersey: Prentice Hall, 1982); Ralph M. Guedeke, *Marketing in Private and Public Non-Profit Organizations* (Santa Monica, California: Goodyear Publishing, 1977); Theodore Levitt, *Marketing For Business Growth* (New York: McGraw Hill, 1974); William Pride and O.C. Ferrell, *Marketing: Basic Concepts and Decisions* (Boston: Houghton Mifflin, 1977); Robert J. Weston, *A Team Approach to Marketing Planning* (New York: American Management Association, 1975).

4. Theodore Levitt, "Marketing Myopia," *Harvard Business Review* (July-August, 1960), pp. 45-565.

5. Kotler, *op.cit.,* p. 66.

6. See, for example: Bruce M. Bradway, Mary Ann Frenzel, and Robert E. Pretchard, *Strategic Marketing: A Handbook for Entrepreneurs and Managers* (Reading, Mass.:

Addison-Wesley, 1982); David W. Cravens, *Strategic Marketing* (Homewood, Ill.: R.R. Irwin, 1982); Douglas J. Dalrymple and Leonard J. Parsons, *Marketing Management: Strategy and Cases* (Third edition, New York: Wiley, 1983); Jon G. Udell, *Successful Marketing Strategies in American Industry.* (Madison, Wisconsin: Mimir Publishers, 1972). For works on marketing strategy in the human and social services, see: Michael L. Rothschild, *An Incomplete Bibliography of Works Relating to Marketing for Public Sector and Nonprofit Organizations* (Third edition, Madison, Wisconsin: Graduate School of Business, University of Wisconsin-Madison, 1981).

7. Jay Conrad Levinson, *Guerilla Marketing* (Boston: Houghton Mifflin, 1984), pp. 26-27.

PART II:
MARKETING RESEARCH
AND TARGETING

Before any marketing plan can be implemented a thorough analysis of a human or social service's environment must be completed. This analysis can be called by different terms such as marketing research, marketing audit, situational analysis and environmental analysis. It includes obtaining firm grasp of the current status of the internal organization and the external environment. The internal area is overlooked many times in developing an audit, but understanding the resources we have in terms of marketing our organizations, the more effective our marketing plans will be. The external environment includes demographic, social, economic, political, cultural and other factors affecting the organization. This evaluation allows the organization to identify market opportunities to pursue and risks to avoid. It also allows for a more sophisticated targeting process before we actually implement our marketing strategies. This targeting process can provide a base to develop concentrated or differentiated approaches to segmentation and targeting. It can prove to be very expensive to initiate an undifferentiated targeting process whereby we try to communicate with all segments of the marketplace and hope we get to the right groups or individuals. Differentiated and concentrated targeting based on the findings of the audit can make the marketing strategies more cost-effective. This is very important as funds become more and more competitive for human and social service organizations. The articles in this section provide some excellent case studies on how marketing research and differentiated targeting can be effective.

WJW

Utilizing a Marketing Audit in Developing a New Service Case Example: Breckenridge Village

John A. Yankey, PhD
Nancy Koury, MSSA
Diana Young, MSSA

Experts generally agree that auditing is the foundation to successful market planning. According to Kotler (1981), the market audit is "a comprehensive systematic, independent, and periodic examination of an organization's marketing environment, objectives, strategies and activities with a view of determining problem areas and opportunities and recommending a plan of action to improve the organization's marketing performance." In brief, Bell (1972) writes that "a marketing audit is a systematic and thorough examination of a company's marketing position."

The purpose of the market audit is to collect and analyze data toward the following objectives:

— To identify problem areas to be corrected.
— To evaluate the overall marketing performance.
— To identify strengths and opportunities to be maximized.
— To understand and anticipate key factors and trends in the marketplace.

Clearly, there is no single "best" market audit method or tool. An audit may take several forms depending on an organization's needs. Different types of non-profit agencies emphasize different areas of investigation. The market audit illustrated in this article contains four components: consumer analysis, internal audit, en-

John A. Yankey is a professor at the School of Applied Social Sciences, Case Western Reserve University, Cleveland, Ohio. Nancy Koury is Coordinator of Case Management Services at Breckenridge Village, Willoughby, Ohio. Diana Young is Program Manager of the Impaired Driver Program at Alcoholism Services of Cleveland, Inc., in Cleveland, Ohio.

37

vironmental analysis, and competition analysis. Through the use of a case example, this article will demonstrate how the market audit can be applied as part of the planning process in the development of a new service.

CASE EXAMPLE

Breckenridge Village is a full-service retirement community located in Lake County, Ohio. It is one of seven such retirement communities in the statewide organization of Ohio Presbyterian Homes. Established in 1922, Ohio Presbyterian Homes' mission is:

". . . in response to the Lordship of Jesus Christ and consistent with His ministry, is to provide full-service, non-profit retirement communities and life enrichment outreach programs. Our communities are dedicated to the enhancement of spiritual, physical and mental well-being, independence, security, and the fullest possible potential for a high quality of life with an environment which promotes human dignity, purpose and self-esteem."

Opened in 1979, Breckenridge Village is the newest facility in the Ohio Presbyterian Homes network. The organization offers a range of care to its residents, including independent living ranch homes, two high-rise assisted living apartments, and a skilled nursing facility. Further, the agency planned to expand its residential base and offer case management and ten other outreach services, e.g., friendly visitors, transportation, and meals-on-wheels, to the elderly in the surrounding communities.

An extensive market audit was conducted by Breckenridge Village, specifically focusing on the development of a case management program. This service was singled out because it posed the greatest financial risk to the organization in that it would require a significant financial commitment.

Case management is a service which provides assessment, linkage, and coordination of services to the frail elder and his/her caregiver. The goals of the service are as follows:

1. To enhance the ability of the older person to remain in the community.

2. To provide support and guidance to the older person and concerned family members.

The market audit was conducted to determine the feasibility, opportunities, and constraints the organization would face in providing case management. The results of the audit were used as a basis for requesting start up funds for community outreach services, including case management, in a proposal to the Robert Wood Johnson Foundation.

CONSUMER ANALYSIS

In a marketing approach, the consumer is the focal point of the planning process. Thus, the market audit begins with an examination of the organization's target consumers—current and potential. The organization seeks to identify its consumers in terms of number, location, demographics, as well as behavior patterns, attitudes, and lifestyles.

In short, data should provide the agency with answers to the following questions:

— Is there a market for this service?
— Is the market substantial and reachable?
— What are the demographics and characteristics of the target group?
— What are service utilization and buying patterns of the target group?
— Are there areas where primary market research is required?

The case management program planners defined the market as individuals 65 years and older living in the western half of the country. The geographic boundaries of this market were selected based on the location of the program facility and the anticipated resources to adequately service this area. Of those 65 years and older, the service specifically targeted the frail—those with physical, mental, and/or social impairments which limit their ability to live independently. This group of elders is traditionally targeted for case management services since they often require multiple health and social services in order to remain in the community.

As shown in Table 1, information from the consumer analysis was the basis for numerous marketing activities of the case management program. For example, based on census data and the planning organization's report, it was determined that a market for case management existed. Further, this market could be segmented into sub-

TABLE 1. CONSUMER ANALYSIS

Source of Information	Type of Information	Uses of Information
Census	. Population 65+ . Demographics (income, age, distribution) . Population projections	. Market identification . Pricing strategy . Market substantiation
Planning Organization Report	. Number of frail persons . Degree of frailty	. Market segmentation . Placement strategy . Market definition
Local Area Agency On Aging Needs Assessment	. Social resources of elderly . Living arrangements of elderly . Health status . Mental health ratings . Unmet needs of elderly . Hospital utilization	. Market segmentation . Demand verification . Promotional strategy . Service design . Decision-making unit analysis
Professional Journals	. Cohort characteristics of elderly . Service utilization patterns . Service needs of elderly . Family caregiving activities	. Service design . Promotional strategy . Decision-making unit analysis . Market segmentation
Unpublished Study of Service Utilization	. Types of services used by frail elders . Levels of frailty	. Service design . Decision-making unit . Market segmentation
Local Human Service Agencies' Annual Reports	. Target group service utilization . Types of services provided	. Market share analysis . Competition analysis . Competitive positioning

stantial and reachable sub-groups. Also, these sources, along with journal articles and the Agency on Aging's needs assessment, provided descriptive information about the characteristics and needs of the target market. These data were useful in developing the program's design and promotional plan. Finally, an unpublished study and the annual reports from local social services agencies offered insight as to service utilization and patterns of the target area's elderly. Uses for this information included further identification of consumer needs, data for the competition analysis, and development of a promotional plan.

The consumer analysis for the case management project also included an investigation of the services decision-making unit. Kotler (1981) has defined five roles in the decision-making unit for any product or service:

Initiator: The initiator is the person who first suggests or thinks of buying the particular product or service.
Influencer: An influencer is the person whose advice and views carry some influence on the final decision.
Decider: The decider is the person who ultimately determines any part or the whole of the buying decision: whether to buy, what to buy, how to buy, when to buy, or where to buy.
Buyer: The buyer is the person who makes the actual purchase.
User: The user is the person who consumes or uses the product or service.

Analysis of the case management decision-making unit included investigation into the following questions:

— How would the older person learn about, gain acceptance of, and make the decision to use this service?
— Who are the significant others in the elder's life who play a part in the decision-making process?
— What are the buying patterns of this market?

Table 2 illustrates the decision-making unit analysis for the case management program—based upon information collected in the preceding section of the consumer analysis. An important finding resulting from this analysis was that older persons are frequently reluctant to initiate services for themselves. Data from several sources reported that many elderly are "too proud" to accept help

TABLE 2. THE DECISION-MAKING UNIT

	Initiator	Influencer	Decider	Buyer	User
Neighbor	X	X			
Clergy	X	X			
Social Service Workers	X	X			
Hospital Discharge Planners	X	X			
Physicians/Health Professionals	X	X	X		
Employee Assistance Programs	X	X		X	
Relative	X	X	X	X	
Daughter/Son	X	X	X	X	X
Spouse	X	X	X	X	X
Guardian	X	X	X	X	
Elder	X	X	X	X	X

from outsiders; too, some elders fear that calling the attention of professionals to their situation may result in institutionalization. Additionally, much has been written about how the frail older person, due to physical impairments and/or social isolation, is often not even aware of existing services.

Because of these factors, the case management planners sought to determine who, besides the elder himself, could act as the initiator of case management services. Research, interviews, and agency care records revealed that the family of the elder, along with physicians, clergy, friends, human services workers, and other significant persons would typically initiate or suggest a service to the elder. Indeed, these individuals also may be involved as influencers, deciders, and buyers as the decision-making roles are not mutually exclusive. Also, the family of the older person may be a secondary consumer of the service.

Results of the decision-making unit analysis were implemented in several marketing activities. First, service buying behaviors and other characteristics of the elderly were incorporated into staff training. Second, because of identified family involvement, an educational component for families was added to the service's design. Third, both target selection and the design of promotional activities were greatly influenced by the decision-making unit analysis of the case management service.

INTERNAL AUDIT

Once the consumer analysis has been conducted, the organization assesses its own capabilities and constraints in meeting the determined needs of the target consumers. Objectives of an internal analysis may include:

— To assess the organization's management capabilities.
— To identify organizational strengths that can be maximized.
— To identify current problems to be corrected.
— To prevent possible future problems.
— To evaluate the organization's abilities in providing services and reaching consumers.

The internal audit is best conducted by a person(s) who is independent and objective. To assure this, an outside consultant may be hired. In some cases, however, a staff member may be assigned to conduct the audit if he/she is sufficiently removed from the consequences of an honest assessment. A consultant often will work with a group of staff members in a team approach to the internal audit.

The internal analysis for Breckenridge Village was first conducted by an outside consultant one year prior to and in preparation for the development of community outreach services, including case management. The analysis was updated and revised by staff members and the chief executive officer a year later as part of the program and market planning process.

The result of the revised internal audit is summarized in Table 3. The audit identified several problem areas of the organization, many of which were remedied since the time of the audit. For example, orientation to the plans for case management and outreach services was presented to the organization's council and residents. In addition, monies were allocated for staff to receive special training to compensate for its lack of experience in outreach service provision. Also, administrative and development staff became more aware of how fundraising would become increasingly difficult as numerous agency needs and programs would compete against each other for limited funds.

Likewise, staff became more aware of how competition for marketing space and attention among organizational departments would also increase. Additionally, the public's perception of the agency as a residential facility would need to be carefully expanded to include

TABLE 3. THE INTERNAL ANALYSIS

AREA	STRENGTHS	WEAKNESSES
Facility	. Beautiful facility . Central location in target area	. Expensive to maintian
Public Perception	. Excellent reputation . Strong community support	. Not known for community services
Staff	. Administration has demonstrated ability for program development and management . Dedicated, hard working staff	. Relatively inexperienced with outreach services
Volunteers	. Excellent track record in volunteer management	. Program recently hurt by lack of coordinator
Fundraising	. Highly successful fundraising	. Facility departments compete for resources . Need to expand relationships
Advisory Council	. Influential and talented members . Active and effective fund-raisers	. Not well informed about plans for outreach services
Marketing	. Technical assistance in marketing offered by local university	. Market orchestration problems
Current Consumers	. Highly satisfied with organization . Active in fundraising and volunteering . Important link to community	. Not well informed about outreach service plans

community outreach services. The organization responded, in part, to these difficulties by creating a marketing/public relations committee consisting of staff members from various departments.

As problem areas of the organization were identified, so were strengths and capabilities. An excellent track record in fundraising, a top reputation in the community, effective volunteer management, and highly satisfied residents demonstrated strong support from the organization's various constituents. The organization was offered (and accepted) technical assistance in marketing from nearby Case Western Reserve University. Further, foundation interest in case management, coupled with strong staff and management, favored the inclusion of the case management program in the proposal.

ENVIRONMENTAL ANALYSIS

No organization exists in a vacuum. Each is continuously affected by its external environment. The external environment is the context in which an organization provides, promotes and distributes its services. In most cases, an organization has limited or no control over environmental factors, yet must be alerted to the threats and opportunities they pose. According to Rubright and MacDonald (1981), "If any organization has any weaknesses, it would be a tendency to overlook the opportunities or obstacles in its marketplace, the external environment." Thus, an important component of the market audit is the analysis of the threats, opportunities and trends in the agency's environment.

Kotler (1981) identifies six components of the "macro environment" which impact an organization's marketing activities. In his model, an examination of political, demographic, economic, ecological, technological, and cultural factors should be incorporated in the market audit. Again, individual organizations may design and structure the environmental analysis with variations based on the needs of the particular agency.

Like the internal audit, the environmental analysis may be conducted by an outside consultant or staff person(s). Board members may be involved in information gathering and should be perceived as sources of information about the community. Other sources of data include the census, local and national newspapers and magazines, professional journals, and interviews with experts.

As seen in Table 4, the external analysis for the case management program covered legal/political, social, demographic, economic, technical and professional trends and issues. These areas were investigated and assessed as to their impact on the development of the case management program.

Several opportunities for the development of case management were found in the external environment. For example, demographics and population trends pointed to a growing target market. Further, DRG legislation and the improvements in medical technology

TABLE 4. ENVIRONMENTAL ANALYSIS

Field	Key Factors	Opportunities	Threats
Political/ Legal	. Local government strongly supports organization . Diagnostic related groupings regulations . Social workers not licensed in state	. Community support for organization . Increased numbers of frail elders in community	. No 3rd party reimbursement . Less credibility
Economic	. Skyrocketing costs of institutional care . Large proportion of middle to upper income elders in target area . Unemployment 12%	. Alternatives to institutionalization sought . Service may be affordable to many	. Cost of service may be prohibitive to some
Technical	. Medical advances have enabled people to survive longer	. Increased need to serve this frail population	. Medical advances may not improve quality of life
Demographic	. County projects 47.5% increase in 65+ age group by 1990 . 95% of elderly living in community	. Increase in target market . Opportunity to maintain elders in their home	. Competition to serve this group likely to grow
Social	. Families provide 80% of care to aging relatives	. Opportunity to support family and relieve some of caregiving stresses	. Families may act as informal "case managers"
Professional	. Trend to community based care . Growing numbers of case management programs nationwide	. Case management program follows 2 national trends in services to elderly	. Competition likely to grow

would likely result in more frail older persons living in the community. Social trends indicated a need to relieve and support growing numbers of family care-takers who, because of jobs, age, children and/or geographic distance, cannot provide all the necessary care themselves. Finally, the increase in the number of case management projects reflect a national trend toward this method of service delivery. While the environment offered many opportunities, several threats to the case management service also existed. These threats were identified in the political and economic fields. For instance, social workers, the primary staff of case management, were not licensed in the state and would not receive third-party reimbursement for service. Consequently, the fees for the service would be paid directly by the user(s). However, a trend toward user fees is developing as human services agencies seek non-governmental sources of revenue. Beyond this trend, the demographics of the target market indicated a potentially large proportion of middle to upper income consumers.

Importantly, other agencies may also recognize the environmental opportunities for case management and develop similar programs that would compete with the case management service at Breckenridge Village.

COMPETITION ANALYSIS

While many human service agencies deny that competition exists, the non-profit sector does have its share of rivalry. Organizations compete for funding, clients, referral sources, qualified staff, community endorsement, and market attention. Indeed, almost all market planning activities are affected to some extent by what competitors do.

Thus, an important step in market planning is conducting a competition analysis. This part of the market audit examines the organization's current and potential competitors. Questions to be answered in the competition analysis may include:

— Who are our current competitors?
— What are their competitive positions?
— What market share does the competition claim?
— Which market segments do our competitors target?
— What are the fee scales, locations, hours, staff qualifications, and funding sources of our competitors?
— Who are our likely future competitors?

Information about the competition may be obtained by several means. Data can be sought through direct requests to agencies for annual reports, promotional materials, and fee scales. Staff and board members of competing organizations may be interviewed. Articles, conferences, and public hearings also provide relevant information. Finally, if data are difficult to obtain by these means, the agency may assign staff or volunteers to call other organizations as potential service users to learn more about the competition.

Table 5 summarizes the competition analysis conducted by the staff of Breckenridge Village in planning for the case management program. For purposes of illustration, six variables were selected from the analysis to demonstrate its use in market planning. The six variables selected were location, fees, related services, market share, market segments, and staff qualifications. At the time of the audit, no other formal case management service existed in the county. Therefore, the competition analysis included all organizations in the aging "industry" focusing on those who may become future competitors.

Results of this analysis aided in refinement and decision-making in several marketing activities, including the selection of a competitive position. For example, the agency's unique location in the west end of the county, its plans to hire a Master's level staff, and the fee-for-service basis all contributed to the formation of a competitive position. Based on these factors, the agency was able to identify its niche in the market as a professional, for-pay service designed particularly for those older persons in the west end of the county. Further, based on a comparison of market shares, the Breckenridge Village case management program chose to aim for a small market share and further position itself as a service where caseloads are low, staff is accessible, and individualized service is possible. Finally, since other organizations provided certain components of case management or offered the service on an informal basis, Breckenridge Village would also claim a unique market position as having the only formal, comprehensive case management program in the county.

CONCLUSION

The market audit is an effective and necessary marketing activity, especially in the planning and development of a new service. As illustrated in the example of the case management program, results from this audit may be utilized in developing the market mix and

TABLE 5. COMPETITION ANALYSIS

	PRIMARY RELATED SERVICE	STAFF	LOCATION	FEES	MARKET SHARE	MARKET SEGMENT
Agency A	Counseling elders and their families	Masters	East	Sliding scales	1%	County elders and families
Agency B	Protective Services	Bachelors	East	No	5%	Abused, neglected, dependent elderly in county
Agency C	Outreach Services	Non-degree	East	No	10%	Persons 60 and over in county
Agency D	Home Health	Nurses and Nurses Aides	East	Yes, supplemented by Medicare	4%	Health impaired elderly
Agency E	Mental Health Services	Bachelors	Border	Sliding scales	2%	Mentally impaired, emotionally disturbed elderly in county
Breckenridge Village	Case Management	Masters	West	Yes, fee for Service	0% Goal: 5%	Frail elderly in western portion of county

competitive position for the service and organization. Importantly, in order for an organization to remain competitive and current, this audit must be updated and revised periodically. Indeed, the organization, the environment, the competition, and the marketplace are likely to undergo frequent and significant changes. A periodic and systematic market audit will help assure that the organization maximizes the opportunities and minimizes the threats these changes bring.

REFERENCES

Bell, M.L. *Marketing Concepts and Strategies.* Boston: Houghton Mifflin Co., 1972.
Kotler, P. *Marketing for Nonprofit Organizations.* Englewood Cliffs: Prentice Hall, Inc., 1981.
Rubright, R. and D. MacDonald. *Marketing Health and Human Services.* Rockville: Aspen Publications, 1981.

A Market Research Analysis of an Adolescent In-Patient Substance Abuse Program

Dennis R. McDermott, PhD

INTRODUCTION

Due to competitive and regulatory pressures marketers of health care services are being forced to develop strategies that are segmentation-oriented. In order to better pinpoint market targets, market research is becoming an increasingly necessary tool as a prerequisite for successfully innovating health care services. The following study illustrates the use of market research, via a combination of focus groups and in-depth personal interviews, applied to test the feasibility of an Adolescent In-Patient Substance Abuse Program as a proposed innovation offered by a private psychiatric hospital.

METHODOLOGY

Data were collected from 30 key referral sources, defined to be those in the community who have the most interaction with adolescents who abuse either drugs and/or alcohol. The respondents comprised three general areas, namely: first, the legal system, consisting of juvenile court judges, probation officers, and court psychologists; second, the educational system, consisting of high school principals, assistant principals, and guidance counselors; and, third, mental health officials, including directors of public clinics and, in some cases, specialists in substance abuse employed by the clinic.

In order to test the study's general hypothesis that an innovative Adolescent In-Patient Substance Abuse Program is feasible and could be successfully marketed, the following specific areas were addressed by the key referral sources:

Dennis R. McDermott, Associate Professor of Marketing at the School of Business, Virginia Commonwealth University, Richmond, VA 23284.

1. What programs or current procedures are they familiar with for treating adolescents who have substance abuse problems and how satisfied or dissatisfied are they regarding these programs?
2. How do they react, in general, to the Concept Statement describing the innovative program and what specific strengths or weaknesses do they perceive?
3. What annual demand do they project for such a program, is the demand likely to increase or decrease, and how confident are they regarding the program's financial success?

The Concept Statement, which was given to each respondent, described the proposed program as a 30 day, in-patient program designed exclusively for adolescents. The program would be chemical-free, would allow for continued educational programs at the hospital, and would strive to involve parents and referral sources with continuous consultation of the adolescent's treatment during both the in-residence period and the post-discharge period, if out-patient monitoring or additional treatment is required.

SURVEY RESULTS

The results of the study will be presented in the same sequence as the three above-mentioned areas addressed by the key referral sources.

Perceptions of Existing Programs

In response to the question: "In past job-related experiences, how are cases involving suspected adolescent substance abusers, where professional help may be necessary, typically handled?", a variety of individuals and organizations were mentioned. In the school-related cases, for example, common procedures included notifying the police if illegal substances were found, and then meeting with the parents, guidance counselor, assistant principal, and school psychologist. A plan of action would then be recommended whereby either: (a) specialists in the mental health field could become involved, for example the Mental Health Clinics in that community; or (b) arrangements for private services would be made, typically out-of-state programs for in-patient treatment.

For court-initiated cases that were deemed low in severity, e.g., first offenses or simple possession of illegal substances, in addition to the above alternatives, adolescent offenders could be ordered to take part in seminars or educational programs on substance abuse aimed at the general population.

Regarding the referral sources' degree of satisfaction with these procedures, approximately one-third of those interviewed said they were satisfied. On further probing, however, they qualified this perception by saying while they were satisfied with the effort or commitment given on the part of the agencies/individuals involved, they were generally dissatisfied (or *very* dissatisfied) with the overall results due to: (a) the lack of availability of specialized adolescent in-patient programs, as it was expressed that out-patient programs are far less effective, and mixing adolescents with adult substance abusers for treatment was very counter-productive; (b) excessive time lags and bureaucratic delays; and (c) lack of parental involvement. The remaining two-thirds of the sample, who indicated an overall dissatisfaction regarding these procedures, generally agreed that the lack of availability of local in-patient programs was the key reason for their response. Many cases were mentioned whereby adolescents were sent out of state to be treated on an in-patient basis, where the effect of these programs was perceived to be questionable since the parents, school officials, court personnel, or mental health professionals, couldn't be directly involved. An additional reason for the dissatisfaction regarding these distant in-patient programs was the concern that any follow-up or out-patient programs that may be necessary after the in-patient period were not feasible.

Concept Statement Reactions

In response to the question: "Do you believe a need exists for a local comprehensive in-patient program oriented to adolescent alcohol/drug abusers, as illustrated by the Concept Statement?", two of the referral sources said there is no real need at this time, and three felt a moderate need exists. The remaining referral sources, representing over 80 percent of those interviewed, responded that a "very definite need" exists for the following reasons:

— demand is high and growing—kids are abusing substances at an earlier age, "hard" drugs are on the resurgence, combination abuse is more prevalent;

— local specialized programs (particularly in-patient) do not exist; have to send adolescents out-of-state; mental health clinics overburdened, not equipped to effectively deal with problems.

A high degree of agreement existed among the referral sources regarding the components of the Concept Statement. When asked if they would be likely to recommend the services of such a program, the vast majority (all but two individuals) said yes. Some reasons given for the overwhelming positive response include:

— I'm willing to try anything, a lot of kids need this badly; nothing but in-patient programs seem to work;
— If program is high-quality, involves parents, and good followup procedures, I would most definitely recommend it;
— Most probably would recommend this but past performance is critical—20 percent success rate would be great;
— Would have no problems recommending this as long as either: (a) the adolescent wants to go; or (b) the threat of jail time as an alternative exists—without this the program probably wouldn't work.

Regarding the issue of separating alcohol abusers from drug abusers, the vast majority (over 90 percent) of the sample indicated no favorable effects would result from doing this. Treating adolescent alcohol and drug abusers in the same program was perceived to be favored due to: (a) adolescents are likely to abuse both substances, and (b) the reasons or causes for alcohol and/or drug abuse are perceived to be similar. The only case mentioned where adolescent drug abusers should be treated separately was that of a heroin addict. A similar high degree of agreement existed regarding the issue of the desirability of separating adolescent substance abusers from adults. Some 80 percent of those interviewed responded that it was "very important" that adolescent substance abusers not be treated with adult abusers since: (a) it is perceived that adults and adolescents abuse alcohol and drugs for different reasons; and, (b) adolescents treated with their peers are much more likely to benefit.

When asked: "What, if anything, would you change regarding the Concept Statement?", the majority of those interviewed replied nothing, and were generally very enthusiastic about its content. Generally, the continuing academic studies feature was viewed very positively as a means of facilitating re-entry. The month-long duration was mentioned as probably being adequate for those adolescents who are experimenting, and would also make re-entry less difficult. Suggested changes regarding the Concept Statement include:

— Time Duration—some one-third of the referral sources favored a more flexible, individualized treatment duration, feeling that 30 days would either "just dry them out", or only provide enough time to identify the problem. Premature discharge is seen as a real concern. At the same time, keeping patients too long, in order to maximize revenues, is also a concern.

— Follow-up/Out-patient counseling—some 20 percent of the sample perceived a need to stress these components more, particularly related to readmission criteria and coordination/cooperation efforts with referral sources; program needs to stress complementary (not competitive) nature to public services.

— Family Involvement—very important to stress treating causes and not just symptoms.

Demand Projections and Confidence Levels Regarding Financial Success

Projecting demand is always a difficult process but when the key referral sources were asked: "In the past year, regarding your job related experiences, how many adolescents have you dealt with whom you believe would benefit from a substance abuse treatment program, as illustrated by the Concept Statement?", a fairly consistent projection of from two to three percent of the high school population emerged. It should be pointed out that the referral sources dealt almost primarily with suburban and not inner-city adolescents. In determining their perceptions as to future substance abuse demand patterns, an almost uniform belief exists that substance abuse among adolescents will increase in the future, particularly regarding alcohol. The rate of drug abuse was perceived by roughly half of the referral sources as being on the increase, while half indicated the rate of drug abuse would stay about the same in the future. In addition, the comment was frequently made that adolescents are abusing alcohol and drugs at a younger age, with the estimate being given by two school officials that for every four or five high school students who would benefit from an in-patient program there would be a pre-high school adolescent who would benefit as well.

When asked how confident they were (high, moderate, or low) that an adolescent in-patient substance abuse program would be financially successful, one-third indicated a high degree of confidence, and two-thirds a moderate or moderate-to-high degree. Some reasons given for these very favorable reactions include:

— Concept Statement—the idea is very sound and with no competition locally combined with a desperate need to refer locally, it's bound to do well;
— In-patient substance abuse programs should start to flourish due to insurance coverage. Parents and school officials are more convinced now that in-patient programs are much more effective;
— Public Programs come and go—very erratic due to funding sources drying up and lack of professional involvement; I'm much more confident a private organization can effectively deliver the necessary services. I'm not bothered at all by their making money in this area as long as the quality is acceptable and some provisions for treating indigent patients (e.g., pro-rated scale, Special Placement Funds) exist;
— There's a crying need for a facility to not only provide in-patient treatment/rehabilitation for adolescent substance abusers, but to also provide guidance/education/leadership for the community's information needs regarding primary prevention, early intervention, recognition of symptoms, etc.;
— Stigma of Psychiatric Hospital—doesn't seem to exist as much now as in the past; operating substance abuse program as adjunct to primary facility seems most appropriate.

SUMMARY

In order to test the feasibility of an Adolescent In-Patient Substance Abuse Program as a proposed offering by a private psychiatric hospital, focus groups and in-depth interviews were conducted with 30 key referral sources representing the legal system, the educational system, and the mental health officials employed by the community. Specific areas addressed by these referral sources included their awareness and perceived satisfaction/dissatisfaction of existing programs, their general reactions to the Concept Statement describing the innovative program as well as their perceived strengths and weaknesses, and finally, their demand projections for the program and perceptions regarding the program's financial success.

Very favorable reactions to the proposed program were given by practically all of the referral sources for a variety of reasons. First and foremost is the fact that this innovative program would be unique to this area, with the referral sources expressing frustration and negative experiences with either out-patient programs or sending adolescents out of state for in-patient programs. In addition, the local programs would allow for far more parental and referral source involvement, thus the causes could better be treated as opposed to simply the symptoms. Other benefits perceived by the referral sources include the adolescent substance abusers would be treated exclusively with their peers and their educational programs could be continued while their 30 day in-patient status existed. Finally, the high confidence of the referral sources regarding the venture's financial success was based on demand projections and the fact that insurance coverage exists in the majority of cases they are exposed to.

As an update, the market research study was a key input to the hospital's being awarded a Certificate of Need for 50 beds for this program. Within three months, 50 more beds were added as the program was operating at full capacity. Within an additional three months, all 100 beds were being utilized. Clearly, the successful application of market research to fill a market void and to generate mutual rewards for the hospital, the community in general, and the adolescents who successfully complete the program, is illustrated in this case history.

Designing a Promotional Tool: Practical Application of Market Targeting and Research: Case Example: Alcoholism Services of Cleveland, Inc.

John A. Yankey, PhD
Diana Young, MSSA
Nancy Koury, MSSA

As social services agencies face a decrease in funding, many aggressively seek new sources of revenues, including an increase in the number of paying clients. To accomplish this, they often turn to marketing. Although marketing is not a "cure-all" for their problems, it does offer benefits to the non-profit sector.

The focus of a good marketing program is the consumer. This is congruent with social services' long-term declaration of being client-centered. With a marketing approach, all aspects of the program package (price, promotion, placement, and product) should be an agency's response to client needs and wants. In this way the consumer becomes the focal point for key decisions in marketing the agency's services.

Two important marketing concepts play an integral part in making the client/consumer the focus of an agency's decision-making: targeting and market research. Rubright and MacDonald (1981) define a marketing target as "any organization or individual that can affect the outcome of the marketing project objective for better or

John A. Yankey is a professor at the School of Applied Social Sciences, Case Western Reserve University, Cleveland, Ohio. Diana Young is Program Manager of the Impaired Driver Program at Alcoholism Services of Cleveland, Inc., in Cleveland, Ohio. Nancy Koury is Coordinator of Case Management Services at Breckenridge Village, Willoughby, Ohio.

59

for worse . . . '' Market targets for social services often include more than just the user of the service. Other consumers include funders, referral resources, supporters (e.g., citizen groups), and/ or legislators.

The other major marketing concept discussed in this article is marketing research. Marketing research can be defined as the organizational activity of systematic gathering, recording, and analyzing the information needed to make planning and implementation decisions relevant to any marketing problem or issue (Flexner & Gerkowitz, 1979; Kotler, 1974; Lovelock, 1984; Rubright & MacDonald, 1981). Data resulting from marketing research do not provide ''magic'' answers for marketing agency services; rather, such data serve as the guidelines for agencies to make better decisions about the program package. Marketing research identifies client needs and preferences on which to base these key decisions instead of management merely guessing what the client needs.

Through the use of a case example, this article will illustrate how one agency program utilized these marketing concepts in developing a promotional tool, the redesign of a program brochure. A brief discussion of the background of the program is followed by the steps undertaken to develop this promotional tool.

AGENCY AND PROGRAM BACKGROUND

Alcoholism Services of Cleveland, Inc. (ASC) is a private, nonprofit United Way member agency. The agency serves Greater Cleveland, Ohio (Cuyahoga County) and the surrounding area. The Board of Trustees decided to address the area of drunk driving in conjunction with a new state law, which mandated 72 consecutive hours in jail or 72 hours in a DWI (Driving While Intoxicated) school in lieu of jail for all first-time offenders. However, the new state law also provided for ''municipal option,'' i.e., it allowed for each municipality to enforce its own DWI code. In ASC's target area, there are 13 municipal courts and 17 mayor's courts, representing a total of 52 judges. The result is a wide range of sentencing of DWI offenders throughout the county and even among the different judges within the same municipal court. With no uniformity of jail sentences, a number of existing DWI schools (varying in length and quality) are utilized in lieu of jail time. This creates a highly competitive environment for the several DWI schools in the county.

ASC's Impaired Driver Program (IDP) offers a 72-hour residential and a 40-hour non-residential DWI program. Both require the participation of a family member or close friend for 16 hours of the program, a unique feature of the IDP. Other DWI programs which require less time involvement for the DWI offender and charge a lower price, present competition for the IDP. It was imperative for ASC's program to implement a marketing plan, including effective promotional tools.

STATEMENT OF MARKET RESEARCH PROBLEM AND OBJECTIVES

After a year of operation, the Impaired Driver Program (IDP) identified the need to redesign its "temporary" brochure to incorporate two aspects: (1) a more professional appearance in the brochure; and (2) update the information with changes made during that year.

As the promotional tool must be consumer-focused, one preliminary step is the identification of the program's market targets. Results of the initial marketing audit, conducted in the product development phase, revealed a decision-making unit made up of several different "influences" and "decision-makers" (depending on which court or judge was involved). These "influencers" and "decision-makers" are judges, probation officers, bailiffs, lawyers, and the offenders themselves (see Figure 1). Thus, written communication, including the brochure, should be targeted at each of these segments (Kotler & Levy, 1969; Rubright & MacDonald, 1981).

Two decisions concerning the development of the brochure rested with management. As part of maintaining a uniform agency image, top management required that several parts of all agency program brochures remain consistent (e.g., agency logo, general agency information, statements required by law and funding bodies, etc.). Middle management (program manager and her supervisor) determined what basic information must be included as a minimum in the brochure (e.g., what, when, price, telephone contact number, etc.). With these as "givens" the question became: What should be the exact nature of the content for the brochure(s) which would target all the various market segments?

This, therefore, became the market research purpose: To develop the most effective brochure, targeted at the various segments of the

FIGURE 1

Decision Making Unit

Figure 1. Decision Making Unit

Police Officer → Arrest

Judge/Defendant → Hearing and Initial Plea

Lawyer → Get Lawyer

Prosecuting Attorney → Prosecutors Hearing

Judge and/or Probation Officer → Enter Plea & Sentencing

Probation Evaluation

Could Plea Bargain Down ← Lawyer / Prosecuting Attorney

Diversion Program

Jail Under New Law

Treatment Program

Jail (Reduced time under Municipal Code)

Jail (For 2nd or Subsequent Offender)

Fines (Ranges from ? to $800)

Good Behavior or Probation → Treatment Program

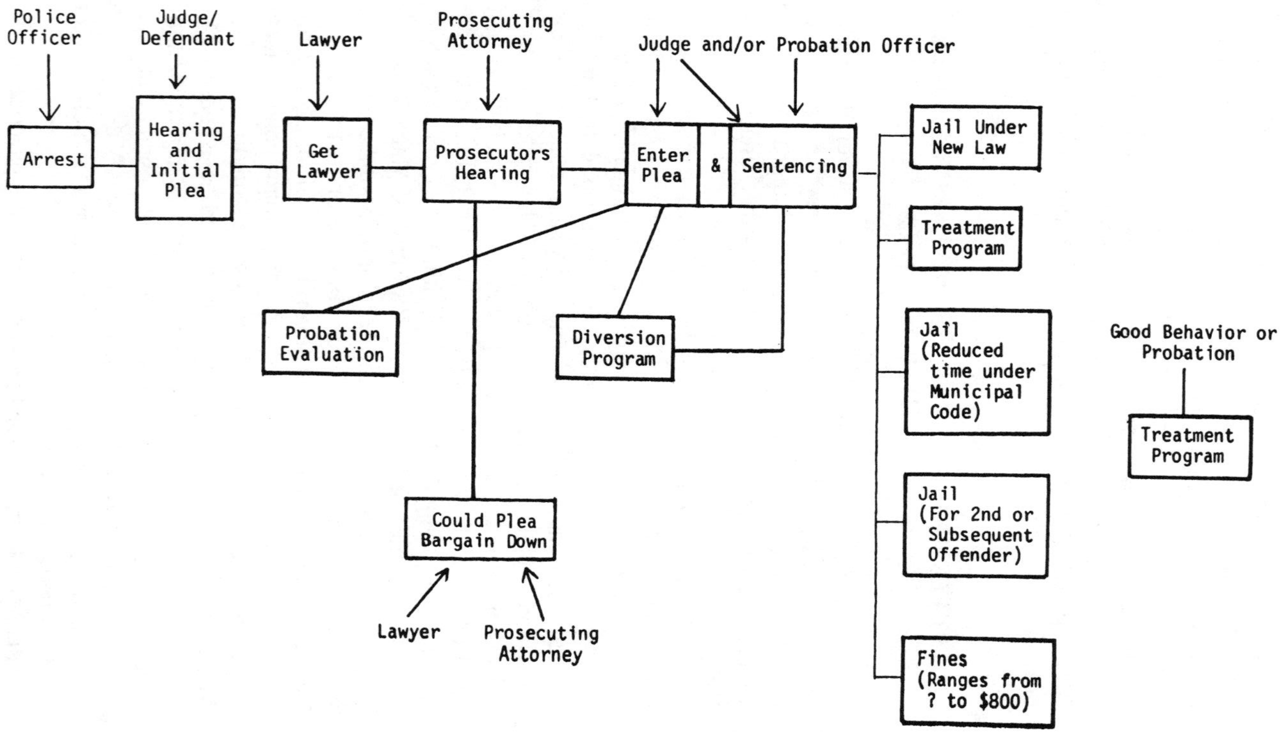

decision-making unit, in order to increase the Impaired Driver Program's share of the market. In refining this to specific market research objectives, clarification was needed on the following:

1. What information is misunderstood or missing in the present brochure?
2. What facts are important to the $\left\{\begin{array}{l}\text{judges} \\ \text{lawyers} \\ \text{probation officers} \\ \text{offenders}\end{array}\right\}$ in their decision-making process?
3. What attributes of the IDP appeal to each segment?
4. What "exchanges"/"benefits" exist for each target segment?
5. Can these different factors be represented in one brochure or are several brochures needed?

SELECTION OF RESEARCH TECHNIQUES AND PROCEDURES

The program manager and her supervisor determined it was feasible to obtain answers to these questions and further, that both primary research (process by which data must be generated) as well as secondary research (data already exist and are available to the program) would be utilized. The following techniques were selected to answer the research objectives:

Objective	Technique	Primary or Secondary
•Information to be clarified	•Key informant interviews with staff members	•Primary
	•Other DWI School brochures	•Secondary
•Important factors in decision-making for:	•Program Reports	•Secondary
•Judges	•Key Informant Interviews	•Primary
•Lawyers	•Key Informant Interviews	•Primary

Objective	Technique	Primary or Secondary
•Probation Officers	•Focus Groups	•Primary
•Offenders	•Client Satisfaction forms	•Secondary
	•Telephone inquiries	•Primary
	•Utilization reports	•Secondary
•Attributes which appeal to various segments	•Same as preceding	•Same as preceding
•Exchange or benefits for each segment	•Same as preceding	•Same as preceding
•One brochure or several	•Analytical step in market research	
	•Management decision	

IMPLEMENTATION OF RESEARCH METHODS

Staff developed an outline of activities required to complete the research and a corresponding task time table. It was decided the program manager of the IDP would have the major role in coordinating and conducting the research activities. Although this raises some question concerning staff bias, operating in a highly competitive environment offered strong incentive for the program manager to remain honest and open in order to formulate the most responsive brochure. Furthermore, two other procedures helped to counter the possibility of staff bias. First, in the latter stage of the development, a draft brochure would be "field-tested," i.e., other agency staff would have input. Second, a consultant team would provide scrutiny over the research procedure. A marketing project team from Case Western Reserve University offered technical assistance through three major tasks: monitored the process to insure validity of activities; provided a "sounding board" for analyzing the data; and brainstormed with staff to develop recommendations.

Staff: The process began with "in-house" key informant interviews. Key staff of ASC were interviewed; namely, those who registered offenders for the program or received initial requests about the program. These staff (professional paid staff, volunteers, and clerical—totaling 5) were asked for their input regarding the brochure. These interviews lasted an average of 15 minutes. Questions covered such areas as:

— Content misunderstood or confusing in the present brochure
— Information currently missing
— Most frequent question(s) asked by service inquirers or registrants
— Attributes of IDP as noted by inquirers

Judges: The next set of key informant interviews was conducted with judges. Program reports were reviewed to ascertain which judges were most actively referring to the program. The program manager attempted to contact 4-5 judges who actively referred to the program and 4-5 who had not yet referred. The key interviews were easily executed by the program manager since her duties as court liaison provided continual contact with the judicial system. Although most judges were available for a personal interview, when necessary interviews were conducted by phone. The sessions lasted between 30-60 minutes and included questions centered around such areas as:

— Typical sentence for a DWI offender
— Conditions appropriate for referral to a DWI program
— Reason for referring/expected outcomes for referral
— Barriers in referring offenders

Attorneys: Attorneys can be significant "influencers" in the decision as to which DWI program an offender attends; therefore, attorneys become a second important target segment. Key informant interviews with attorneys were somewhat more difficult to execute. Several attorneys from the agency's Board of Trustees were interviewed, as well as two attorneys who called for their clients to request information about the program. Typically, attorneys would not afford as much time as the judges. Interviews lasted 15-30 minutes and included such questions as:

— How did you hear about the program?
— What is the most important factor(s) in selecting a DWI program for your client?

— What aspects of the program do you feel are most appealing to your client?

Probation Officers: A third target segment for research activities was the probation officers. A focus group offered the opportunity for input by 6 probation officers from different municipal courts. Eight probation departments (varying in size and representing demographically different municipalities) were initially contacted by phone, followed by a formal written request to those who responded favorably. A skilled volunteer (Master's level student intern) served as the group facilitator, rather than the program manager, to enhance the probation officers responding candidly. Some questions were similar to those asked the judges and lawyers, but additional ones were added concentrating particularly on referral procedures (as probation officers are often the court's channel for completing assignment forms with offenders). The focus group lasted approximately 90 minutes, following which those participating were provided lunch.

Users of the Service: Input from the actual user of the service (DWI offender and his/her family member) was gained in several ways. At each month's session, the participants (offenders) and the co-participants (family members) complete evaluation forms on the final day of the program. The evaluations consist of rating general areas of the program and responding to open-ended questions. Monthly summaries of these evaluations reflect the group's ratings as well as all written comments. In reviewing the summaries, reoccurring comments provided insight as to what attributes of the program seemed especially appealing to the participants and co-participants; what areas of the program warranted further explanations; what areas created negative feelings; and clues as to misconceptions formed prior to attending the IDP.

Secondly, for a two-week period, those receiving initial requests were asked to make note of reoccurring questions from the offender and/or the family member. Thirdly, utilization reports were reviewed to determine what reasons potential users offered for not completing registration. Those aspects identified as least appealing to offenders could then either be minimized in the brochure, turned into a positive attribute of the program in the reader's eyes, or more fully explained to provide a satisfactory rationale for the program's methods.

ANALYSIS OF DATA

The next step was to analyze the information gained through these research activities. Analyzing was primarily the task of the program manager, her supervisor, and the development officer (whose graphic skills and creativity were to aid in the brochure design and wording, and who also offered an objective perspective). As previously mentioned, the marketing project team from Case Western Reserve University also offered an objective review of the data. The authors will not attempt to reflect all the information gained through the analysis techniques. However, examples will be presented to illustrate how these activities answered the market research objectives. Most evident in the feedback were those items commonly misunderstood or missing in the temporary brochure:

— Program's status as to state certification
— Session content
— Eligibility requirements
— Requirements of co-participants
— Hours for attendance (residential vs. non-residential vs. family)
— Location

Commonalities noted among the factors employed by the "decision-makers" included the need to meet 72 hours (in some courts); what courts are utilizing the school; and cost. The analysis led to important findings regarding the perceived program benefits/ exchanges for each target group:

Judges: •Concerned with over-crowding jails
                   •Reduction in recidivism
                   •Need to answer to community
                    voice (e.g., MADD)

Lawyers: •Need state-certified school
                   •Least costly and restrictive

Probation Officers: •Easy method of referral
                   •Thorough assessment of probationer's drinking

Participant: •Comfortable facility, privacy
                      •Non-threatening experience
                      •Caring staff, who "treat you like
                      human beings"

APPLICATION OF FINDINGS

Based on the findings from the market research activities, a draft brochure was designed and "field tested" with agency staff and the marketing consultants, as well as members of the general public. The brochure integrated data regarding currently missing or misunderstood information with the necessary and factual information needed by all those seeking to learn about the program. The feedback on readability and accuracy resulted in few changes.

As a result of the field testing, it was noted that the initial draft did not expound on the various benefits or desirable attributes for the different market segments; rather, it made general statements which did not adequately cover these specific points. Through further discussion with staff and the technical assistance team, three inserts were designed for the brochure. One insert was designed to target members of the judicial system (judges, bailiffs, probation officers, lawyers) which allowed for each segment to be targeted separately on this insert (see example in Figure 2). A second insert was targeted at the individual participant. It serves as an informal discussion with the offender to inform him/her in more detail what happens there and to create a caring, accepting tone (see excerpt from insert in Figure 2).

A third insert was designed to target family members. This attempts to recognize the feelings a co-participant holds in being required to attend the session; and, further helps him/her to understand what is expected of a co-participant during the session. Because this component is the most misunderstood, the desired outcome is to lessen co-participants' anxieties and initial hostilities. (See Figure 2 for excerpt from this insert.)

MONITORING AND EVALUATION

No market strategy is complete without a plan for monitoring and evaluation. Semi-annually, the IDP's statistics are reviewed by its program staff and management of ASC. This promotional tool will be reviewed as part of that process. Additionally, feedback from the

FIGURE 2. EXCERPTS FROM THE INSERTS OF IMPAIRED DRIVER BROCHURE

TO MEMBERS OF THE JUDICIAL SYSTEM:

Judges - By sentencing the DWI offender to the Impaired Driver Program you can:

. provide an alternative to overcrowded jails.

. reduce recidivism

. provide viable answers to your community's questions about drunk drivers and their treatment in the court system.

Attorneys - By referring your client to the Impaired Driver Program you will offer them:

. a state-certified program recognized by the courts of Cuyahoga County

. an educational experience which can be long-term positive benefits

Probation/Parole Officers - Referral to and involvement with the Impaired Driver Program offers many benefits:

. you secure an easy method of referral

. you receive an assessment regarding your probationers/ parolee's drinking

. you have access to three-way conferences and useful follow-up information which can save you time and effort in your casework

TO THE PARTICIPANTS:

It is a shock to be convicted for a DWI offense. If this is your first time through an IDP you must be wondering what's in store for you ...

The setting is comfortable and safe. The food is good and the surroundings combine the atmosphere of a hotel setting and an educational workshop ... There will be films, lectures, group discussions and private sessions with caring and skilled professionals.

TO THE FAMILY:

"Why do I have to come to this program? I wasn't the one caught drinking and driving!"

Most family members involved in the Impaired Driver Program ask this question, usually with a bit of anger and upset feelings ...

You will see films, hear lectures and have many chances to ask questions. You will meet others who have to face the same problems and worries and learn how others cope.

target segments will be solicited on an on-going basis as staff receive service inquiries from offenders and their attorneys. The IDP staff meet quarterly to review program issues. An item for discussion will be any feedback received on the brochure, particularly if staff have observed an attitude change by the family on the initial day of the program. Finally, on an annual basis, evaluation forms containing questions concerning the brochure are mailed to judges and probation officers for their feedback.

CONCLUSION

Many agencies do not fully embrace the practice of marketing, especially marketing research. The reasons cited for this are usually lack of skilled staff, inadequate time available and/or no monies allocated for such activities. It is true that some marketing activities may require seeking outside marketing expertise. However, as Lovelock (1984) notes in his reference to market research, "The goal of marketing research is to reduce uncertainty to tolerable levels at a reasonable cost." In other words, expending dollars in the present can keep the agency from spending unnecessary dollars on activities which do not effectively address the problem. Without the implementation of targeting and marketing research in the case example, an ineffective brochure would have been developed which ignored the essence of the marketing principle—the exchange value for its market targets.

Furthermore, this case example illustrates that marketing research does not always have to be complicated and time-consuming. Most research activities fit into the daily tasks of the program manager; therefore, limited additional time expenditure is required on the part of the staff. All activities with the target segments served as additional visibility for the program. With very little money expended, the agency was able to avoid wasting money on an inadequate promotional tool. Instead, two marketing concepts—targeting and market research—were invaluable in the development of an effective IDP brochure.

REFERENCES

Flexner, W.A. & Berkowitz, E.N. Marketing Research in health services planning: a model. *Public Health Reports,* November-December, 1979, *94*(6), pp. 503-513.
Kotler, P. *Marketing for non-profit organizations.* Englewood Cliffs, New Jersey: Prentice-Hall, Inc., 1975.

Kotler, P. & Levy, S. Broadening the concept of marketing. *Journal of Marketing*, January, 1969, *33*, pp. 10-15.

Lovelock, C. *Services Marketing*. Englewood Cliffs, New Jersey: Prentice-Hall, Inc., 1984.

Rubright, R. & MacDonald, D. *Marketing Health and Human Services*. Rockville, Maryland: Aspen Systems Corporation, 1981.

PART III: MARKETING STRATEGIES: MARKETING MIX, POSITIONING AND SALESMANSHIP

Marketing strategies are the broad actions that an organization can implement to satisfy the original goals and objectives of their marketing plan. The basis for developing marketing strategies is diverse. Strategies can be based on the marketing mix whereby characteristics of the PRODUCT, PLACE, PRICE, PROMOTION and PEOPLE related to the organization. The first article by Rosanna Pribilovics at the Family Service Agency of S.F. was developed especially for *HMQ* to demonstrate how these five components of the marketing mix can form the base of successfully marketing a human service agency.

When developing strategies it is important to understand the barriers that have to be overcome in marketing select human and social services. This stigma can be overcome if strategies follow a thorough planning process. The second article in this section describes this process for overcoming a stigma when marketing mental health services. Understanding how to overcome this stigma allows the organization to better position itself into the minds of the clients. Positioning the organization as unique in comparison to other human and social service agencies allows for a competitive advantage.

The training of social workers typically does not include any strong management courses, especially in the areas of marketing. One key marketing strategy that can benefit human and social service managers is salesmanship. The third article outlines for the reader the importance of salesmanship and marketing strategies for the typical social service manager and relates it to the advertising aspect of marketing.

WJW

Marketing Mix Case Study: Family Service Agency of San Francisco

Rosanna M. G. Pribilovics

INTRODUCTION

Marketing has become one of the most important tools of managing today's social and human service agencies. Marketing allows the human service administrator to communicate effectively internally and externally with the different publics with whom the agency serves and interacts. It can be a valuable tool for making human service agencies more effective. This article describes the variety of successful marketing strategies which have been used to market one of the oldest and most established human service agencies in California, the Family Service Agency of San Francisco (FSA/SF).

Brief History

In 1889, San Francisco was an untamed and intemperate city. It was characterized by a high incidence of child abuse and neglect, poverty, and very limited amounts of social service assistance for the local citizenry. In response to the need for coordinated provision of social services and proliferating charitable agencies, the predecessor to FSA/SF, Associated Charities, was formed. This organization and its successors were involved in such activities as the 1906 earthquake relief, great flu epidemic of 1918, development of foster homes and adoption programs, and the relief efforts related to the Depression. In 1938 the Family Service Agency of San Francisco

Rosanna M. G. Pribilovics is Associate Director of Family Service Agency of San Francisco.

This article was written in collaboration with Ira Okun, Executive Director of Family Service Agency of San Francisco.

was formed, became incorporated and joined the Family Service Association of America. It also became a member of the Community Chest which now is known as United Way. In 1944 it merged with the Children's Agency of SF to form the Family and Children's Agency of San Francisco. The agency changed its name for the last time and became known again as the Family Service Agency of San Francisco in 1958.

The agency has been located in San Francisco for ninety four years. Kitty Felton, the first director of FSA/SF, commissioned Bernard Maybeck, the famous California architect, to specifically design a building for the agency on Gough Street in 1928. The building was built by a grant from the Prescott Estate and is characterized by an aesthetic and functional urban but Spanish Colonial style. It has been declared a historical landmark in San Francisco. (See Figure 1.)

Through the years FSA/SF continues to meet its mission of providing services to families and children under stress, promoting the general welfare of the total community, advocating for the elimination of conditions that cause family life to deteriorate, preventing unnecessary institutionalization of family members, preventing dependency on public welfare systems, and aiding families to promote the physical, mental, and emotional development of their children.

The agency has continued to expand its service base. Today, it provides such services as child abuse prevention, case management for the developmental disabled, family counseling, aftercare for chronic mentally ill, geriatric care, child care, comprehensive care for pregnant teens and teen parents, counseling for Japanese and Chinese populations, advocacy for nursing home residents, foster grandparent program, senior companions, parental stress line, group counseling, respite care for high risk parents, family violence programs, and others. These services have been developed to meet the current health needs of the county of San Francisco, without regard to financial constraints. An affirmative action policy exists for all sectors of the agency's clientele. FSA/SF consists of twenty-five programs organized into three major departments.* The agency has a budget which exceeds five million dollars per year and employs approximately two hundred people. Funding is derived from a variety of sources including United Way, private foundations, public agencies, fees, and individual donations.

---

*See Organizational Chart (Table 1).

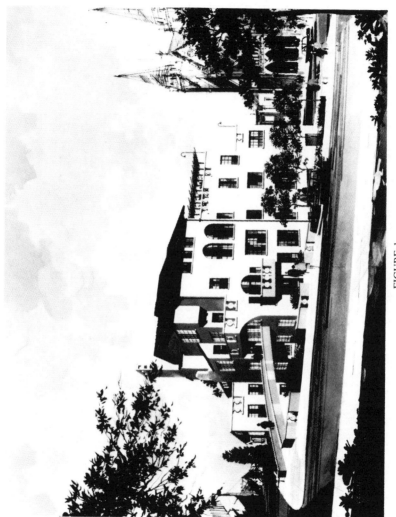

FIGURE 1.

77

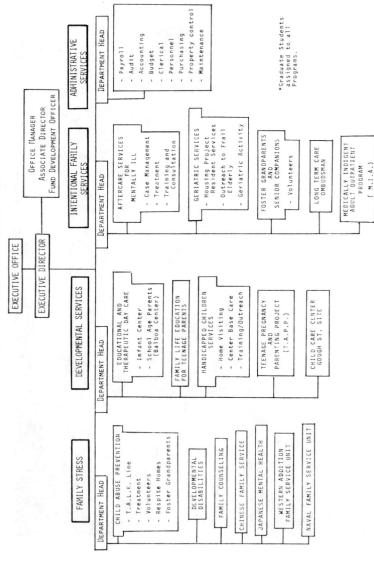

FAMILY SERVICE AGENCY OF SAN FRANCISCO – 1984

TABLE 1.

MARKETING STRATEGIES AS APPLIED
TO THE MARKETING MIX

An excellent way of presenting the wide variety of marketing strategies that FSA/SF has utilized through the years is to group them into the components of the marketing mix. These components include the Product, Place, Price, Promotion and People. The strategies are applicable to multiple types of non-profit social and human service organizations. They are systematically organized for easy reference.

Product

A quality human service organization must have an attractive service which offers value to the client. These values have to satisfy the unique health needs of the client. A product/service portfolio must be established which outlines the service mix which most effectively serves these health needs of the population.

Family Service Agency of San Francisco offers a variety of services in its portfolio to meet selective health needs of the community and to diversify and remain financially viable. The bottom line is to serve humanity and in order to do so, FSA/SF has had to approach this need by effectively managing the organization. FSA/SF has used the concept of opportunity management which emphasizes (1) the development of organizational mission, goals and objectives, (2) market opportunity identification, (3) strategic planning for taking advantage of these market opportunities, and (4) effective implementation.

For example, the Teen Pregnancy and Parenting Project (TAPP) at the FSA/SF followed this systems approach to its development and implementation. The original director, Kitty Felton, was involved in trying to get better services for pregnant teens and teen parents. For ten years, she began a successful campaign to close a foundling hospital with the highest infant mortality rate in the city. This activity satisfied the organizational's mission of providing services to high risk families and the organizational goal of meeting the needs of teen parents. There is a growing incidence of teen pregnancies and teen parents during the past few years. FSA/SF had the foresight to identify this health need, or market opportunity, many years ago. The passage of federal legislation and monies in 1976, presented a funding option to implement the market opportunity.

Using FSA/SF's historical precedence and existing small teen parent infant program, coordination was established between social work, education and the health community. FSA/SF became the fiscal agent and spokesperson of the teen parent service community. The market opportunity now changed to require the offering of comprehensive services such as medical, nutrition, education, day care and career planning. This allows the teen parent to become economically independent, lowers the risk of children being born with abnormalities, and potentially reduces the likelihood of child abuse. In collaboration with the San Francisco School district and thirty other human service agencies, a methodology for providing these services was developed.

Under the direction of the current Executive Director, Ira Okun, a strategic plan was developed through the years for providing this wide scope of services to this group. This plan included identifying the problem, soliciting funding sources, establishing staffing requirements, lobbying for effective legislation, educating the community as to the existence of the problem, networking with other human service agencies for the provision of comprehensive services and the prevention of duplication, and obtaining input from community groups, coalitions, advisory committees, users of the services and other relevant sources.

FSA/SF has effectively implemented this program through the networking of multiple private and public human service organizations such as SF Unified School District, SF Dept. of Social Services, Florence Crittendon, Children's Home Society, Legal Services for Children, SF Public Health Dept., etc. All of these organizations are components of TAPP. Their complementary resources are collaborated to meet the needs of the pregnant teen and teen parents. The program has been successful in serving over 500 clients with excellent independently documented results and generating millions of dollars in cash and in-kind programs.

This program is a good example of a marketing strategy which emphasizes the importance of linking the historical and current mission of the human service organization. It also exemplifies how the agency does not operate in a vacuum. The agency provides services by obtaining input from the community for opportunity identification. This means identifying a social need, planning for satisfying this need, and implementing programs designed with input from other human service organizations.

The reputation and longevity of the agency is a key attraction to clients. Being one of the oldest agencies of its type in California and known for quality services provides for a strong base of referrals. The foundation of longevity for this successful agency has been the ability to create and implement the service mix. This success reflects a marketing sensitivity to understanding the people it serves, their needs, and an ability to network with other human service organizations to provide these services. The networking aspect is vital for preventing duplication, containing costs, and being able to adequately allocate scarce human service resources.

Place

A key aspect of developing a marketing strategy is related to access to the service, location, availability, waiting times, etc. FSA/SF has consistently attempted to market their services through a strategy of lowering the barriers for client access. FSA/SF has never had a lack of clientele. There are waiting lists for several programs. However, client access to the services is important whether the agency is trying to attract new clients or not. FSA/SF considers access to be an important consideration in planning for the delivery of services.

It is reflected by having various sites depending on the need of the clientele, such as the Chinese Counseling Program. This program is a service which is physically located in the Chinatown section of San Francisco. The residents will not come for services at the main agency. Therefore, the service must be provided where it will be needed and utilized. The closer a service is to the source the greater the likelihood of being used by its target population. Other examples include FSA/SF's Family Stress Programs based at the Naval Station at Treasure Island and the Army Base at Presidio of San Francisco.

Another example of the place component is improved access to public transportation. For example, the agency is physically located between two main bus lines, within walking distance to BART, and in close proximity to a major freeway. One service actually possesses funding for bus passes for clients. Another one provides a van for transportation to and from the agency.

The hours of operation are a key ingredient for the place component. For example, FSA/SF operates an average of approximately twelve hours/day. This allows for evening counseling appointments and group meetings. The agency permits other organizations to use their facilities for optimum utilization. Another example is the twenty-four hour parental crisis line, the TALK Line, which provides telephone counseling to high risk and abusive parents. The Child Care Center operates from 7am to 6pm. Working, low-income, parents from the local community drop their kids off before going to work and are able to pick them up after a normal work day is completed.

The flexibility of how services are provided is a characteristic of the place component. Some services are provided entirely in the home. For example, the Developmental Disabilities Unit and the Home Education Program For Handicapped Infants delivers its services in the home. If necessary, other services such as counseling can be provided in the home, senior public housing, nursing homes, and board and care homes depending on the need of the case and funding source.

FSA/SF has a good screening methodology to make sure the client is linked to the needed service. Assistance is given to triage clients to the most appropriate FSA/SF and other community services. Examples would be referring battered women to a shelter, clients to Dept. of Social Service for entitlements, and children to St. Luke's Hospital's Speech and Learning Center for evaluations. An effective agency will keep up-to-date with information about current community services. This is especially important in large metropolitan areas where human service turnover is high.

In the counseling department, an intake worker is available during working hours for drop-ins or telephone counseling. An individual or family in crisis can obtain assistance immediately on this basis. In addition, for continuing clients receiving service, efficient appointment systems is vital for long-term relationships.

The way in which services are provided in term of access makes a difference in the success of the service. This ensures that the client is able to use the service more effectively.

Price

The pricing component of the marketing mix is an important factor for human service organizations. FSA/SF's policy to pricing is that no client will be turned away due to their inability to pay. The agency does not rely solely on fee-for-service. Instead, revenues are derived mainly from private and public contracts.

FSA/SF's success is based on its pricing abilities. The key form of pricing for FSA/SF is the charge to funding sources based on the efficiency of operations. A large part of FSA's funding is derived from government sources. An RFP will be issued by a government agency and interested human service agencies will competitively bid for the program. FSA/SF has been able to submit strong bids because a broad base of funding has been developed, thereby controlling indirect costs. For example, in 1978 the agency's indirect costs were 18% of total costs as compared to 15.5% in 1984. The use of professionally trained and supervised volunteers also assists in lowering costs. Because of today's competitive market for financial resources, FSA/SF will selectively take risks in bidding for contracts at a rate lower than the actual costs of operating the program. At a later date, the full value of the programs can be recouped as refunding occurs for successful operating programs. In addition, United Way of Bay Area is an important funding source. Its flexible dollars allows FSA/SF to bid for programs which are weakly funded by other sources. FSA/SF uses its discretionary dollars to buttress public funded services. Therefore, the client receives the service they need without concern for their ability to pay.

There are two methods used in determining fees for FSA/SF services. FSA/SF funded services such as the Parental Crisis Line, Mothers' Group and Single Parent Support Group have no direct charge to the client. A sliding fee scale developed for FSA/SF's Counseling Services has an hourly charge based on the client's income and family size. In this case, the scale ranges from no charge to forty-five dollars. The second method depends on public funding requirements, i.e., the Universal Method of Determining Ability To Pay (UMDAP). It is a formal scale used by community mental health system and is based on monthly income and number of dependents. Those programs funded by Community Mental Health, such as the Japanese Mental Health Program, Aftercare, and Geriatric Program, are required to use this fixed fee schedule. Another public funding system is the California State Department of Education Fee Schedule, i.e., Child Care Center. Fee-for-service does restrict the clientele an agency can serve in terms of income constraints.

From a marketing perspective, it is important to be competitive through exploring a wide range of funding sources, operating as efficiently as possible, communicating these different pricing methods effectively to clients, and to establish a strong network of support from financial and political resources. In today's competitive marketplace, an agency cannot depend on any one funding source. Funding and pricing analysis is an on-going component of marketing.

Promotion

Promotional strategies relate to the methods of communicating with the different publics with whom an agency serves or interacts. Promotion typically includes such areas as public relations, personal selling, sales promotion and publicity. These strategies usually encompass soft-sell, hard-sell or educational approaches. Most human service agencies utilize soft-sell and educational methods for promotion. This is especially true when a large proportion of agencies are not in need of more clients. When this is the case marketing becomes an effective communication tool to enhance relationships with staff, boards, other human services in the community, governmental agencies, and clients. Many human service agencies dependent on fees and insurance compete heavily for clients and orchestrate their promotion to obtaining clients. Most promotion for agencies which do not need more clients, as exemplified by FSA/SF, is related to (1) improving and sustaining the image of the agency in the community; (2) attracting Board and advisory members; (3) developing strong relationships with current and future funding sources; (4) creating an effective internal communication link with staff; and (5) reinforcing the referral network with other community human service resources.

FSA/SF utilizes public relations for informing the community about their programs and services. This is accomplished through the use of brochures, flyers, newsletters, annual reports, speeches and other strategies initiated by management staff.

Brochures/Flyers: The agency maintains a regularly up-dated group of brochures developed for specific purposes. These include a low-cost mass distribution brochure about the entire agency; an additional detailed brochure describing the entire agency for use with professionals; individual program brochures to target specific publics such as the elderly, teen parents, and Chinese population; and program announcements/flyers for distribution.

Newsletters/Annual Report: Three newsletters describing specific services and/or fund raising activities are distributed to thousands of current and potential donors. These donors can include individuals, select corporations, foundations, board members, and staff. An annual report highlighting the prior year's activities and outlining future agency goals is also distributed to the donor base.

Speeches: The management staff make speeches to community and business groups for advocating issues, educating on available services, and for fund raising activities. Individual program staff will occasionally give presentations on specific programs and current social issues.

Meetings: The executive director or delegates are active members in many community organizations and associations. These include such organizations as: Teen Parent Coalition, SF United Way Executives, Mental Health Contractors of SF, Mental Health Advisory Board, Mayor's Sexual Trauma Advisory Committee, Elderly Abuse Prevention Consortium, Developmental Disabilities Council and many other key community groups. The executive director is expected to participate in activities that are in the best interests of the clients we serve or the fiscal needs of the agency.

Fairs and Special Events: Whenever financially feasible, the agency sets up information tables and booths at community events. These include such activities as: SF County Fair, Independent Living Exposition, Children's Network Conference, and various United Way campaign events.

Working with Board: The Board of Directors plays a vital role in marketing the agency in terms of image-making, networking, fund raising, and public relations activities. FSA/SF employs a fund development officer who works closely with the board on these activities in conjunction with the executive director. The fund development officer acts in the capacity of educating and training the board of directors for fund raising needs and their role and responsibility in fund raising and public relations. An example of a fund raising event in association with the Board of Directors is Operation Home Run. This event is a baseball game between media personalities and politicians. Tickets are sold to the general public and proceeds are designated for the child abuse prevention programs at FSA/SF. Besides actual funds, the event strengthens support and publicity for the entire agency.

Public Service Announcements/Advertisements: Close ties are maintained with local media for educating the public about select services through public service announcements. Advertisements are placed in newspapers to educate select target groups about services. Posters are placed in public transportation, child care centers, laundromats, supermarkets, and other high-visibility avenues. Stuffers are also placed in utility bills and diaper services for select programs. Telemarketing is utilized, for example, in relation to the annual fund raiser, Operation Home Run, for contributions. Telemarketing has the potential to be a key marketing strategy for human service agencies in being able to communicate with a large group of people quickly and at relatively low cost.

People

The most important strategy for marketing an agency is the effective utilization of the agency's human resources. This is evident by the important roles that the board, administrators, staff, and volunteers play in marketing FSA/SF. The Executive Director of FSA/SF, Ira Okun, is the main planner and coordinator of marketing activities for the agency. Through his leadership during the last seven years, FSA/SF has expanded significantly in terms of programs offered and financial base. If a human service agency is to be effective in its marketing activities a strong executive director is essential. The Executive Director at FSA/SF administers the agency through his management team which consist of a controller, department heads, project directors, associate director and developmental officer.

The backbone of delivering quality services to the public is the staff of FSA/SF. The staff consists of such professionals or direct service personnel as family counselors, social workers, psychiatrists, psychologists, child care workers, volunteers, and various administrators. Every staff member is a marketing representative of the agency. It is important for each staff member to be educated and believe in the mission and goals of the agency and their individual programs. In-house training and effective newsletters are important strategies in enhancing the marketing role of each staff member. For example, FSA/SF is currently developing an internal newsletter to meet these needs.

A major human resource for most agencies are volunteers. These volunteers are involved at FSA/SF in telephone counseling for the TALK Line, tutoring in math and reading in the Chinese program, advocating for seniors in nursing homes through the Nursing Home Ombudsman Program, being an adjunct parent for children in hospitals, respite care homes, and child care centers, and offering to be companions to the home-bound frail elderly. All of these volunteers are formally trained by the agency for their assignments. There are as many volunteers as paid staff at the agency. There is also an internship program for graduate students from local universities. These interns provide monitored services in a clinical setting. The volunteers and interns provide a cost-effective, quality mode of delivery. They become marketing representatives for the agency in their interractions with clients, staff, and other community resources. FSA/SF has strong ties with the community through the use of specialized advisory groups. These groups allow for community input and a base for agency networking. Some of these groups include: Navy Family Service Center Advisory Group, Elderly Abuse Prevention Task Force, Nursing Home Ombudsman Advisory Group, and Board and Care Advocacy Group. The members of the groups include representatives from the general public, organizations, and professionals in their specialized field.

CONCLUSION

FSA/SF is a fine example of a human service agency which has been effective in sustaining and expanding its base despite tumultuous economic times. Marketing has played a vital role in this success with attention being given to the five Ps of the marketing mix: Product, Place, Price, Promotion and People. There are some valuable lessons to be learned by human service administrators in terms of effective marketing. Since the majority of human service administrators and clinicians are not trained in marketing, it is important to begin to integrate this tool into their management repertoire. Marketing is a much broader and useful management tool and rarely recognized as such by the majority of social and human service providers. As financial pressures become more acute in the human service marketplace, it is important to adapt and strategically plan for the future. Managers need to be active rather than reactive to changing environmental conditions. Comprehensive marketing methods can assist human service agencies in taking advantage of opportunities. However, marketing must be integrated along with financial, economic, and human resource management techniques for effective strategic planning. Effective strategic market planning has to take into consideration these components of the marketing mix. As an agency increases in their professionalism, the more sophisticated strategic market planning must become.

Fighting the Stigma: A Unique Approach to Marketing Mental Health

Gregory D. Nelson
Mary Beth Barbaro

One of the frequently expressed concerns of mental health professionals has been the overwhelmingly negative image associated with their business. This oft repeated concern is shared universally by agencies, centers and clinics regardless of size or geographic location. Major categories differentiating mental health care continue to be misconceived by our publics; they approach mental health problems with a combination of detachment, fear and trepidation. The plain fact is that we have an image problem, frequently labeled stigma.

FIGHTING THE STIGMA (FTS), introduced by SERCO in 1983, was an interstate pilot designed to concentrate on the problems of stigma as well as promote mental health care. FTS involved five participating mental health organizations, each with unique market characteristics. These facilities—one in Indiana, Illinois, Kentucky, Ohio and Oklahoma, represented an excellent cross-section of the various publics served by mental health care organizations. For example, in Lawton, Oklahoma, a rural environment dominates while in Galesburg, Illinois, the environment is tempered by a neighboring metropolis. A similar comparison applies to mid-size Dayton, Ohio, traditionally an excellent test market within the sixty-minute markets of both Columbus and Cincinnati. To complete the strategy, a more metropolitan environment was represented by the Louisville participant, and a middle-American population in Fort Wayne, Indiana.

FIGHTING THE STIGMA was based on two central goals. The first was to create a *favorable impression* toward the utilization of

Gregory D. Nelson is Executive Director and Mary Beth Barbaro is an Associate of SER-CO, Inc., a marketing and promotion firm specializing in mental health.

mental health services and programs *among specific consumer groups.* Coincidentally, each participating mental health center was promoted as a qualified provider of services. Furthermore, in order for this campaign to have long-term potential for mental health care in general, FTS was conceived as a pilot whereby these locations were viewed as test markets. Thus, the second goal was to test the feasibility and potential impact of a similar campaign expanding to the national level with extended target markets.

One of the major influences in planning FTS was the fundamental, yet critical procedure defining the needs to be met, determining the groups who possessed the needs, and creating a viable program in response to their needs. SERCO coordinated the marketing strategy which applied key marketing principles and focused on two target markets identified by the participants. The strategic plan was based on three key success factors:

1. SERCO's pivotal coordination and evaluation role;
2. The multi-media campaign itself, which incorporated a central theme, a consumer-specific message and participant endorsement; and
3. The sharing of developmental costs.

In scheduling objectives for FTS, SERCO categorized them as either "Planning" or "Implementation." The *Planning* objectives included program development, the marketing strategy, pre-production planning, cost analysis and research/evaluation criteria. *Implementation* objectives executed the aforementioned Planning objectives, including such stages as production, distribution, testing and evaluation.

PLANNING AND IMPLEMENTATION

The Planning objectives as they were accomplished are grouped in the following categories: Preliminary Tasks, Consumer Research, Production and Distribution.

The first stage, Preliminary Tasks, included writing and issuing the Prospectus which provided the necessary background information, the marketing plan, schedules and financial criteria. Subsequently, the participants were recruited and lists were compiled for potential target markets.

Full use of the target market concept was utilized by coupling knowledge of demographic characteristics with an understanding of the consumers' basic motivations. Since another contingency in reaching a target is understanding the willingness to purchase the service, such issues as social pressure, physical location, pricing and competing interests were also considered. Thus, not only the need for and interest in the service was considered, but also disposition and *ability to pay*. Subsequently, two target markets were identified based on the participants' responses. The next stage, Consumer Research, defined these audiences.

Target Market A (henceforth, TM-A) consisted of young, married couples, aged 26 to 39, with one spouse professionally employed full-time and the other most likely employed at least half-time. TM-A couples had young children or teenagers and lived in middle to upper-middle income, residential neighborhoods. They were active in church and community activities. Problem areas for TM-A included career development/job stress, separation/divorce and family stress.

Target Market B (henceforth, TM-B) consisted of older, married couples aged 55 to 69, recently retired professionals. Their children were grown and not living at home; TM-B couples resided in middle to upper-middle income areas and were involved in service groups and community organizations. Problem areas for TM-B included loneliness and depression brought on by aging, life style changes as well as separation and divorce.

Extensive consumer research was compiled for both TM-A and TM-B to ensure that the programs developed would be responsive to their needs. Pre-production focus groups were conducted to glean crucial data about the attitudes of the audience and their degree of interest or lack of interest. The panels, comprised of 8-10 representatives from each respective target market, were established to determine the most beneficial copy concepts, images and themes. A consumer-oriented message was then produced for each target market, TM-A and TM-B, and subsequently aimed at the markets via *paid* television spots, full color print materials (i.e., posters, brochures) and radio PSAs.

In the Production Phase, rough texts were analyzed including several possible approaches and themes. All FTS materials centered on a unified them—"Counseling. The best thing you'll ever do for yourself" (see Figure 1); with the underlying premise that people hesitate to seek professional counseling for fear that others might

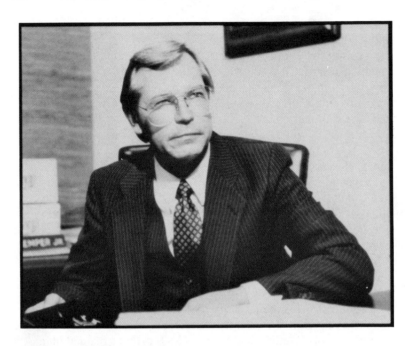

I did it.

**Counseling is the best thing
I've ever done for myself.**

Yes, I've had professional counseling. I'll admit it. At first it was hard to ask for help. I was afraid people would think I was crazy. But the counselor explained to me that my problems were normal signs of stress. With help, I learned to recognize these signs. I learned to find ways of reducing my stress, and now I'm happier with both my job and my family.

From my own experience, I know you're not crazy just because you need help. You're crazy not to ask for it.

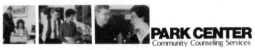

PARK CENTER
Community Counseling Services

Call 482-9111 24 hours a day

FIGURE 1

think they are crazy. In order to impact the target markets, the materials were highly specific and consisted of vivid color graphics, dynamic headlines and believable copy as tested by focus groups, consumer panels, etc.

In the final Planning stage, Distribution, the best media buys were solicited in each designated market area (DMA) from the top-ranking television stations. After a thorough analysis relative to the intended audiences (i.e., TM-A and TM-B), the best media package was purchased.

Since positioning is also a key success factor in print distribution, the need to analyze the distribution sites was critical. The abridged roster in Figure 2 lists the "most likely" distribution sites for the posters based on the consumer profiles of TM-A and TM-B. These sites were established as guidelines to enhance the potential message/market interface and to avoid indiscriminate circulation.

Once these Planning objectives were accomplished, the Implementation Phase began including production and distribution of the materials as well as testing and evaluation. The Implementation Phase of FTS was unique since few cooperative or long-range media efforts have gone beyond the project "theme" and targeted specific consumer groups at the individual participant level.

THE EVALUATION PHASE

The FTS strategy consisted of an evaluation phase designed to analyze the project relative to mental health. Extensive pre- and post-test telephone surveys (Total N = 5,406) were implemented to ascertain attitudinal background regarding the general public's conceptualization of mental health services and their providers. In addition to attitude assessment, reach and impact studies analyzed recall and/or change in recall for each participant and the services provided. To insure objectivity and statistical validity, the results were analyzed by both SERCO and Paragon Opinion Research (an independent research firm).

Distribution Locations for Print Materials (Abridged List)

Target Market "A" (Age: 26-39)	Target Market "B" (Age: 55-69)	Sites Applicable to Both Markets
Office Complexes	Senior Citizens Centers	Recreation Facilities
Public/Private Schools	Medical Buildings	Public/School Libraries
Physical Fitness/Health Facilities	Retirement Communities	Public Buildings (e.g., Post Office)
Company Bulletin Boards	Cafeterias	Churches
Convention Centers	Pharmacies	Grocery Stores
Shopping Malls	Nutrition Sites	Banks
Athletic Events	Transportation Systems	Parks/Zoos
Travel: Hotels/Motels	Beauty Salons/Colleges	YMCA/YWCA
Educational Programs/Events	Historical Sites	Fine Arts Centers: Music/Dance
Theatres	Housing Projects	Museums
		Drama/Art

FIGURE 2

The survey results reveal that demographic characteristics play a key role in the decision whether to seek professional counseling. For example, it is evident that older people are generally less tolerant of the idea of counseling, with those over 55 most resistant. To illustrate, 69.80% of the respondents in the 65 and older category *agreed* that "When a person is having a problem, it's best for him or her not to think about it but to keep busy with more cheerful things." Conversely, only 33.36% of the respondents in the 18 to 24 age group agreed with that statement. Even more noteworthy, only 7.9% of the respondents over 65 *strongly* agreed that going to a counselor is nothing to be ashamed of; in contrast, a far greater 24.65% in the 24 to 34 age group chose this more weighted response. These results are not surprising because throughout the project, respondents over the age of 55 consistently were uncertain and resistant to the concept of counseling.

In general, as the level of education increased, tolerance to the idea of counseling increased as well. For example, 92.26% of the respondents with some post-college education *disagreed* with the statement, "Very few people would benefit from counseling," while only 63.69% of the respondents with less than a high school education disagreed with the statement. Furthermore, in response to the statement, "Everyone needs help at sometime in his life, and going for counseling is nothing to be ashamed of," 33.9% of the post-graduates chose the more weighted response category of "Strongly Agree" while only 11.84% of the respondents with less than a high school education chose that category. One interesting tendency was that as education increased, the percentage of respondents choosing the "Don't Know/No Answer" response decreased. This may be due in part to a clearer understanding of and comfort with the concept of counseling.

The most significant research finding is the confirmation of the premise on which FIGHTING THE STIGMA is based—stigma and the concomitant image problems. Regardless of age, education or marital status, the bottom line is that more than 90% of *all* respondents believed that "Some people who want to go for counseling *don't,* because they're afraid that people might think they're crazy." It appears that within the communities studied, individuals who may want to seek counseling are concerned with potential stigma.

In the post-test surveys there was a significant increase in positive ratings of mental health services in general, as well as in name recognition of the specific mental health centers. Not unexpected, the increase was most significant among the specified target markets (i.e., TM-A and TM-B). In addition, several centers experienced an increase in utilization during the campaign, many of whom referred specifically to the television commercial.

Furthermore, the evaluation indicated a clear correlation between favorable responses and exposure to media. Figure 3 illustrates this point while showing the consistency of results in all five DMAs (designated market areas).

Not only does the media source affect overall response, but there is also a direct relationship between the number of different types of media encountered and the strength of the rating. The synergistic benefit of utilizing more than one medium to obtain a desirable response is illustrated in Figure 4. The "Very Favorable" response is the most weighted response. In this category, each medium has a positive influence; nevertheless, the affect on those who were exposed to all three media sources is far more significant with a 37.89% *increase* over those without media contact. Although a favorable impression does not necessarily mean a willingness to go to a facility, the favorability measure will play a key role in any choice decision which might be made in the future. Furthermore, relative to Goal One set forth in this pilot, the evidence clearly demonstrates the capability "to create a *favorable impression* toward the utilization of mental health services and programs among specific consumer groups."

FIGHTING THE STIGMA produced decisive findings which verify the potential and positive impact of a well coordinated media campaign. To the knowledge of this author, never before has mental

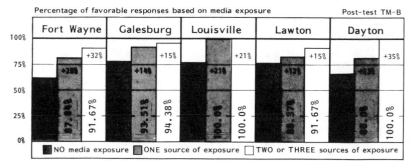

FIGURE 3

Respondents' general impressions of participating centers comparing those with
NO media, ONE source or ALL sources of media exposure.

Response	Question: Thinking of everything you've read or heard about (the participating center) overall, would you say your impression is Very Favorable, Somewhat Favorable, Somewhat Unfavorable or Very Unfavorable?		
VERY Favorable	Exposure to Radio only 7.4%		
	Exposure to Print only 18.5%		
	Exposure to Television only 40.7%		
	Those with exposure to ALL media sources 64.51%		
Very/Somewhat Favorable (Combined)	Those with ONE source of media exposure 88.33%		
	Those with exposure to ALL media sources 94.20%		
	There were a total of 107 UNfavorable responses (Very/Somewhat). The following graph illustrates the variance between NO and ALL media exposure categories.		
Very/Somewhat UNfavorable	4.7%		
	(Those with exposure to ALL media sources)		

0% 5 10 15 20 25 30 35 40 45 50 55 60 65 70 75 80 85 90 95 100%

FIGURE 4

health advertising been so comprehensive. Where previous efforts to promote mental health care have relied heavily upon public service announcements and "free" publicity, FTS implemented paid television spots and full color posters and brochures. Press releases and PSA's were used but not relied upon as the sole source of exposure.

The data compiled provides conclusive evidence that although counseling may be an acceptable "concept" in 1984, the willingness to seek help is tempered by stigma and uncertainty. Stigma is real; before a positive change can be made in the extent of acceptability of mental health services, we must face this reality.

As result of FIGHTING THE STIGMA, the foundation for a systematic, long-term project has been established. It is upon this success that work has begun on FIGHTING THE STIGMA II. FTS II presents a unique strategic plan which responds to the problems of stigma while promoting specific organizations and their services.

FTS II STRATEGY

The FTS II strategy is predicated on three related findings from the pilot:

1. *You can impact your publics and improve your market position*—This point is critical to the daily activity in a mental

health organization. At the onset of a personal problem, the consumer evaluates various resources which might be considered helpful. When consumers evaluate those choices, the "position" a mental health care provider holds is generally a last place position, or frequently, it is not even considered in the initial decision process. By applying the principles of identification advertising in the FTS strategy, that position can be improved. As a result, our marketing plan is designed to vie for position among the target markets, as well as competitors, with as little disruption in an organization's day-to-day activity as possible.

2. *The extent of impact depends on the receptivity of the target market*—Whether or not consumers decide to seek mental health services is related to demographic characteristics and experience; for example, in the pilot two major influences on the choice decision were age and education—NOT the cost of services. The FTS strategy includes identifying the market that has the most potential to understand an organization's services and their benefits.

3. *Predictions for growth in the mental health profession are positive*—The extent of the exposure to situations related to mental health is expected to grow, along with realized benefits. For example, our response to the high technology all around us was the evolution of a highly personal value system to compensate for the impersonal nature of technology. The result was the new self-help or personal growth movement, which eventually became the human potential movement. The implication for the mental health profession is apparent. This trend is supported by noted social forecaster, John Naisbitt, the author of *Megatrends,* who writes that "the more high technology around us, the more need for human touch." Regardless of the therapeutic techniques mental health professionals espouse, human touch is still their priority . . . and their expertise. The FTS II strategy is founded on that belief.

One precedent in the FTS pilot was the use of paid advertising and the scheduled release of related materials; the success of the FTS marketing plan was not contingent upon the negligible benefits of preemptible public service time, nor upon any single medium. The pilot verified that mental health organizations can improve their market position by reaching specific audiences, and one guarantee for that market/message interface is via paid television. In the revised strategy for FTS II, the potential reach and impact of the paid advertising is greatly enhanced because of the following modifications:

A. In place of a split media buy as occurred in the pilot, FTS II, will feature consecutive weeks of television broadcasts.
B. Rather than shifting the market emphasis in mid-campaign, this strategy will concentrate on one major target market throughout.
C. With pre-testing schedules one month prior to implementation, the distribution of related materials is planned for two week periods before and after the flight dates.
D. Unlike the third and fourth quarter media buy in the pilot, this strategy is based on a first quarter media buy when bonuses and other significant benefits result in more coverage per dollar spent.

THE FTS II CONSUMER

In order for the FIGHTING THE STIGMA II marketing strategy to have successful impact, it is necessary to have a clear understanding of the consumers involved. By studying consumer needs, characteristics and behaviors, the market can be divided into well-defined segments. The goal then, is to identify a target whose high-incident potential will maximize the possibility of eliciting consumer response to the media campaign and its message.

Consumer groups can be formed on the basis of geographic variables (regions, cities), demographic variables (age, income, education), psychographic variables (life styles, activities, interests) and/ or behavioristic variables (problems recognition, benefits sought). In addition to these characteristics, it is also important to analyze the target audience's media habits. This can increase the potential reach and impact of the FTS II media campaign.

After a thorough analysis of consumer research, a profile for the FTS II target market has been compiled by coupling knowledge of demographic and psychographic characteristics with an understanding of consumers' basic motivations. Subsequently, a consumer group has been selected for whom the message will be tailored, with the intent of strengthening the impact of the target market/message interface.

Briefly, the first determinant for the FTS II target market (hence-forth, FTS II-TM) was age; males/females 29 to 45 years of age. Similar to the FTS pilot, FTS II-TM is comprised of career-oriented professionals in the middle to upper-middle income bracket. In general, FTS II-TM feels good and positive about life. However, the need to be successful and avoid failure, to preserve one's self-concept and the need for social approval quite often are identified as problem areas. When needs go unfulfilled, they produce pressure and tension. This tends to increase and worsen the problems of everyday living, causing emotional instability. Basically, problems arise when needs are unable to be satisfied.

In general, three most relevant problem areas for FTS II-TM are work-related problems, parent/child conflicts and personal identity problems.

Since mental health services are considered "unsought," the readiness stage of FTS II-TM is awareness of services but disinter-est in seeking them. Primarily, this is because of the negative at-titudes and beliefs about mental health care. FTS II-TM attitudes show resistance to change to the extent that beliefs are anchored in their conception of self-worth. Thus, the FIGHTING THE STIG-MA II strategy is designed to promote new images rather than trying to change old ones.

Because of the unsought nature of mental health services, the aim of the media message is memorability versus direct response. In order to build a positive, long-range image, non-overt appeals (e.g., slice of life) will be used. Thus, messages will be designed in such a way that they are directed toward the consumer whose life style, dispositions and need states are consistent with the above FTS II-TM profile.

TEST MARKETING FTS II

In implementing the FIGHTING THE STIGMA II marketing strategy, feedback from consumers representing the target market is crucial. The information that is obtained from test marketing can in-crease the potential reach and impact of the FTS II media campaign and its message.

A widely used research tool, test marketing involves introducing a new marketing program into authentic consumer settings to learn how the target market will react to the product/service. In this regard, SERCO decided to test market the FTS II strategy in a situation resembling one that will be faced in the full-scale launching of the media campaign.

A complete advertising and promotion campaign has been implemented in a test market which is similar to markets that will be targeted in the FTS II project. This will glean primary data indicating how well the campaign materials and message perform and what revisions are needed, if any. SERCO is undertaking this measure in order to achieve a more reliable forecast of the FTS II strategy as well as pre-test the marketing plan and subsequently enhance the potential message/market interface.

CONCLUSION AND SUMMARY

Although stigma is a problem, there is a definite solution. As this material suggests, an impact can be made by targeting various markets. Since these markets have either positive, negative or neutral impressions of their local mental health organizations and the related services, knowing their *rating* of the organization and the services helps to identify the most likely targets.

Advertising can directly affect the strength of that rating in a positive direction. The *extent* of that affect, whether it's a change in attitude or level of recognition, will depend on the continuity of the message, the channels of communication and synchronization of distribution.

In addition, the degree of impact is contingent on how amenable the target audience is to the message. In the case of mental health, the lower level of acceptability presents an even greater challenge. The FIGHTING THE STIGMA project takes on the challenge with a marketing plan that is necessary because our *publics* say it's necessary. And it can work because, again, our *publics* say it works.

The supporting evidence is more than just an increase in name recall and favorability factors. The supporting evidence results from any project which has been planned and implemented with the *consumer* in mind. Finally, the supporting evidence is clear in the interest and contributions of each participant in the FIGHTING THE STIGMA pilot, as well as the twenty-four mental health organizations in nine states scheduled to participate in FTS II.

The full evaluation of this pilot (122 pages) is available. If you would like more information about FIGHTING THE STIGMA, its follow-up, FIGHTING THE STIGMA II, or marketing mental health services in general contact:

Gregory D. Nelson
SERCO Marketing
600 Wayne Avenue
Dayton, Ohio 45410
800/654-2400
In Ohio call 513/223-0012

The Salesmanship
of Social Work

Constantine G. Kledaras

This paper will consist of two parts. Part I will give a general framework discussing an overview of marketing. Part II will deal with a specific focus, that is, relating one aspect of marketing—advertising—to the profession of social work.

The writer begins by making some postulates or premises. *One* has to do with the marketing concept which states that the satisfaction of consumer needs is a central concept of marketing. To quote:

> The function of marketing is to study and interpret consumer needs and behavior and to guide all business activities toward the end of consumer protection. (Rewoldt, Scott, Warsaw, 1977:5)

Two, the marketing concept is no longer perceived as being exclusively relevant to the business or for-profit sector of the economy. The potential utility of marketing principles beyond the business sector has prompted a broadening of the marketing concept. To quote:

> Marketing is the analysis, planning and implementation and control of carefully formulated programs designed to bring about voluntary exchanges of values with target markets for the purpose of achieving organizational objectives. (Kotler and Zaltman, 1971:5)

Given this definition, the marketing concept and marketing strategy has become potentially applicable to organizations in the

Constantine G. Kledaras, Professor, Department of Social Work and Correctional Services, Carol Belk Building—312, East Carolina University, Greenville, NC 27834.

not-for-profit sector that include colleges, museums, churches and hospitals (Kotler, 1979). The identification and understanding of consumer needs and attitudes thus become a necessary condition of effective marketing (Quelch, 1980).

A frame of reference and definition of the marketing concept deals with the formulating of a marketing strategy which traditionally involves the framing of policy in four areas of decision making: (1) the product policy; (2) the pricing policy; (3) the distribution policy; and (4) the communication policy. An internally consistent plan of action in each of the four policy areas is known as the marketing mix and constitutes a marketing strategy. This definition has gained widespread acceptance as being applicable to the marketing of products (Kotler, 1972) and services (Rathmell, 1974) in both for-profit and the not-for-profit sectors of the economy (Kotler, 1979). It is important to note that distinctions are made between marketing and public relations. According to some writers (Clarke, 1978; Quelch, 1980) marketing is not equivalent to advertising. Advertising and public relations are merely two of the tools, along with personal selling and sales promotion, which are available to the marketer in designing his (her) communication policy. This distinction is important to point out because of the controversy that prevails in our own profession concerning the use of public relations as a technique or tool for improving the image of social work (NASW Newsletters, 1978-80).

The utility and application of marketing strategy to other professions and disciplines has been a source of study. For example, in the marketing and health care industry a number of articles have discussed the application of marketing management and strategy in health care organizations (Lovelock, 1977; Fryzel, 1978; Garton, 1978). In this context a perspective is viewed whereby:

— the "seller" is the health care organization
— the "product" is the preventive intervention or service offered
— the "consumer" is the person who responds to the offer—the patient or potential patient.

A similar analysis and application to social work becomes evident:

— the "seller" is the social work organization
— the "product" is the service offered
— the "consumer" is the person who responds to the offer—the client or potential client.

There are many barriers to successful marketing of which widespread inadequate understanding among professionals of marketing strategy and the design of effective communication programs seem to this writer to be the most pronounced. Justifications for its usage include cost-benefit or cost-effectiveness, rise in inflation, greater governmental regulation, exposure to commercial companies who use marketing concepts and who are suppliers to the for-profit as well as to the not-for-profit sectors of the economy, and the increasing emphasis on consumer orientation philosophy. Despite inflation, costs and increased government regulation, there appears to be a trend toward services that are being more and more tailored to the needs of the consumers (Title XX, third-party vendorship, private practice).

Thus, to summarize Part I of this paper:

1. The central concept of marketing was established—which is the satisfaction of consumer need;
2. The function of marketing was discussed in terms of its broader and more inclusive meaning which incorporates the profit as well as the not-for-profit sector;
3. The definition of marketing was made in relationship to the four policy areas which serve as the marketing mix and constitute the marketing strategy;
4. A distinction was made in terms of equating marketing to advertising or public relations; and
5. Barriers to successful marketing and justification for its usage were presented.

Next, the writer will turn to Part II of this paper which deals with the specifics of the relationship of the topic to social work. It is in the communication policy of the marketing strategy that advertising has its greatest impact for social work as will be demonstrated in the pages to follow.

For some time this writer has attempted to answer for himself the compelling question which has plagued him for some time—that is, what is it that is missing in a social worker's repertoire? The observation made throughout the years is that there appears to be a missing ingredient germane to social workers. This observation has troubled this writer for some time. After many years of practice inclusive of the mental health field and social work education a search was begun in an attempt to unravel this mystery and seek answers to this perplexing and disquieting question. This inquiry led the writer to the discovery that of the many positive characteristics and traits that social workers possess the salesmanship quality or characteristic is the mystery ingredient that appears to be missing. Many interpretations in terms of personality, sociological and psychological theories can be posed as explanations. This section of the paper will not attempt to deal with such discussions as causal explanations. The writer will leave this exploration to the reader for his (her) own speculation. The paper will attempt, however, to highlight features in salesmanship and advertising that are similar to social work and if carefully scrutinized and addressed could enhance the skills of the social worker. The gist of this paper, therefore, is made in the form of an appeal to the reader to question and challenge this premise and to stimulate further thinking and discussion.

In reviewing this question, the writer turned to the literature to seek answers. The writer reviewed over thirty-five catalogues and bulletins from graduate schools and undergraduate programs in social work. Of the catalogues reviewed the writer found no course offerings or descriptions pertaining to salesmanship or advertising in the schools of social work. This led the writer to ask the question—why is salesmanship or advertising lacking in the training of social work? Was the issue basically related to a lack of knowledge in this area by social workers? Was it an issue related to the meaning and connotation of salesmanship and advertising, and its implication and usage in the business field? Did it relate to the nature of salesmanship and advertising and the evils of advertising? Lastly, is there such an incompatibility in philosophical orientations between and within the two fields of practice? In attempting to seek answers to these questions an investigation of the literature in advertising was made. An analysis revealed that there are many essential features inherent to good advertising that seem pertinent and relevant to the development and practice of social work. Some of these features will be highlighted in the discussion to follow.

MANAGEMENT OF PEOPLE AND AGENCY

One of the key features that appeared to recur in the literature on advertising dealt with the matter of management of people and agency (Groesbeck 1972: 46-220; Carson, 1958). A sincere, frank and honest appraisal and appreciation of people and their efforts seemed to be a significant factor to successful advertising (Cardamone,

1959:13-17; Stebbins, 1957:35-52). Timing and praise were important salient features in the provision of high standards of service (Bedell, 1952: Chapter 12; McClure, 1950:275-278; Stebbins, 1957:52-86). The stress and importance given to this matter is exemplified in the following quotation:

> Probably there never was a business as highly personal as advertising. It depends for success on individual work, inspiration, enthusiasm. It makes use of temperamental, highly strung individuals to where a word of *praise* in the proper spot means far more than money. (Groesbeck, 1964:1)

An index to good advertising dealt with the actual delivery of services. A sign of a good salesman was one who kept his (her) promises (Stebbins 1957:73-75). A weakness was seen in the person who could not deliver what he (she) promised. Vitality and freshness were emphasized as needed for continued good salesmanship. The maintenance and upkeep of the human factor was seen as necessary to good advertising. "Job Burnout" or "The Burnt Out Syndrome" was evident in advertising as in social work (Maslack 1978; Kahn 1978). According to one author:

> And it is precisely because you add yourself that it is so important to cultivate resources within yourself; to keep regenerating the only battery that regenerates itself—the human mind (Stebbins 1957:5). . . The point is: to be a better advertising man—get away from it. (Stebbins 1957:53)

High ethical standards seem imperative for successful advertising (Carson 1957:95-99; Groesbeck 1964:13-25; St. Thomas 1956: 18-32; Barton 1958: Chapter 14; Bedell 1952: Chapter 15). Responsibility, reliability and restitution were emphasized in terms of agency ethics (Groesbeck 1964:34-35). The act of delegating was another important element to good advertising. To quote:

> Above all, the head of the agency must know how to delegate. The clients don't like the management of their accounts to be delegated to juniors, any more than patients in hospitals like the doctors to turn them over to medical students. The pursuit of excellence is less profitable than the pursuit of bigness, but it can be more satisfying. (Ogilvy 1963:16-17)

CREATIVITY

Another salient and recurring theme found in the literature for good advertising was the subject of creativity (Carson 1958: 140-143; Gottschall and Hawkins 1959:224-231; Stebbins 1957: 3-40; McClure and Fulton 1964: Chapter 9; McClure 1950: Chapter 14). It appears that for successful outcomes in advertising creativity is not only important but an essential element. According to Frank Barron:

> Creative people are especially observant, and they value accurate observation (telling themselves the truth) more than other people do.
>
> They often express part truths, but this they do vividly; the part they express is the generally unrecognized; by displacement of accent and apparent disproportion in statement they seek to point to the usually unobserved.
>
> They see things as others do, but also as others do not. . .
>
> They are born with greater brain capacity; they have more ability to hold many ideas at once, and to compare more ideas with one another—hence to make a richer synthesis.
>
> . . . They are by constitution more rigorous and have available to them an exceptional fund of psychic and physical energy.
>
> Their universe is thus more complex, and in addition they lead more complex lives. . . .
>
> They have more contact than most people do with the life of the unconscious—with fantasy, reverie, the world of imagination.
>
> They have exceptionally broad awareness of themselves. . . .
> (Barron 1958:164-165)

This excerpt on creativity is *a propos* to advertising as it is to social work as evidenced in the literature. The danger and foe to successful advertising is conventionality as it leads to a dissipation of talent and mediocrity. One author expresses his concerns by stating:

Thinking takes thought. Few of us think . . . Thoughts take time. That's why thought is hard work. And that's why we spend much time and thought avoiding the idea of thought . . . Advertising today is suffering from the luxury of mediocrity—a luxury business cannot afford. (Stebbins 1957:3)

He further observes that:

A healthy segment of American advertising today is modern in thinking and ingenious in interpretation; but for most part there is too little copy—and too much copy-cat. Too much *imitation* and not enough innovation. And if we can't *innovate* let's at least renovate. (Stebbins 1957:6)

Another outstanding leader in the field expresses his concerns in a similar fashion. He views advertising as a business of words but, also, sees advertising agencies comprised of men and women who cannot write. The majority of men and women who are responsible for advertising today, both agents and clients, are conventional. The business community wants remarkable advertising but turns a cold shoulder to the kind of people who can produce it. The kind of talent needed is most likely to be found among nonconformists, dissenters, and rebels. Original thinking goes beyond reason and his criticism of the business men are incapable of original thinking because their imaginations are blocked (Ogilvy 1963:19-21).

Creativity, hard work, an open mind and an ungovernable curiosity are seen as essential qualities for successful advertising (Cardamone 1959:1-14). To quote:

Advertising is arrived at by instinct and a kind of subtle unselfishness: I mean the capacity to step outside of one's own narrow view and foresee and forefeel the emotions of others. (Bedell 1952:20)

But to be *truly* successful in the business world the magic ingredient to success is the ability to sell what one creates. The ability to *sell* or the salesmanship quality appeared to be the outstanding characteristic of good advertising and was the predominant and outstanding factor to success in the literature:

An advertising man is a man who takes *facts* and translates these ideas into *emotions*; translates emotions into *people*; translates these people into *sales*. . . . To move products you must move people. (Stebbins 1957:3-52)

Another expert concludes:

. . . . it is useless to be a creative original thinker unless you can also *sell* which you create. Management cannot be expected to recognize a good idea unless it is presented to them by a good salesman. (Ogilvy 1963:21)

Thomas D'Arcy Brophy defines good salesmanship as "salesmanship with a sense of responsibility" (Stebbins 1957:52). Perhaps this same observation and criticism can be applied to social workers. Social workers thrive on authenticity, autonomy, individuality and creativity (Rapaport 1968:139-161) but apparently lack that special ingredient identified with good salesmanship. It may stem from a lack of basic knowledge and skill in salesmanship. A corollary, however, to creative salesmanship for successful advertising is strong leadership (Groesbeck 1964:19-37). Ogilvy feels so strongly about this point that he makes the assertion that no creative organization can produce a great body of work unless it is led by formidable individuals. He views few of the great creators or innovators in advertising possessing bland personalities. In fact, he views the great creators as cantankerous egotists, the kind of men who are unwelcomed in the modern corporation (Ogilvy 1963: 21-23). This analogy might be applied to social workers as they, too, can be viewed in a similar fashion. Representing the conscience of society social workers are often viewed as willful, capricious, and unwelcomed by the modern corporation which created them (society).

CLIENT RELATIONSHIPS

Another recurring theme throughout the literature dealt with client relationships—that is, how to get clients and how to keep clients (Barton 1958: Chapter 13; Stebbins 1957:40-160; Freeman 1957:1-30; Blumenthal 1972: Chapter 8). Proper human relationships are a must to the success of the advertising agency (Groesbeck

1964:46-210). Good listening is conducive to good advertising. According to one author, "one good strategem which seems to work in almost every case is: get the prospect to do most of the talking" (Ogilvy 1963:34). A caution or warning to aspiring managers of agencies is made. By virtue of the nature inherent in the position of manager or keeper of people, the position carries with it certain dangers. It can be viewed as a traveler on the edge of a precipice. It can be stormy and have its ups and downs. It takes a strong secure person to fulfill this role (Bedell 1952: Chapter 12). There is little room for insecure frightened people. As one author so aptly states:

> The imagination to conceive, the faith of labor, the courage to date—this is the great trinity of advertising success. And the greatest of these is courage. It simmers down to this: If you won't dare, you won't do. (Stebbins 1957:159)

Client turnover can become a problem. To keep clients and reduce client turnover, the agency must devote the best brains to the services of clients (Barton 1958:234-251). Another technique conducive to good client relationships is maintaining contact with and about clients at all levels (Groesbeck, 1964:257). This can become a troublesome area for some agencies as they become larger. This type of problem is depicted as "the insulation pitfall." A reason why top level people in big corporations tend to practice this "insulation tendency" or "arm's length policy" with their agencies is that they dislike the whole business of advertising because it is so intangible and speculative (Ogilvy 1963:58-59). The speculative and intangible nature of advertising is described in the following excerpt:

> Advertising deals with the alchemy of the human heart and mind. That's why you can't reduce it to a mathematical formula. You can't measure the human equation with test tubes or tape measures, with millines or micrometers. (Stebbins 1963: 45)

This same criticism can be applied to social work. Social work receives much criticism because it is not an exact science and much knowledge remains in the realm of the non-scientific, the non-explainable, the non-rational (Rank 1958: 1968; Robinson 1949). Sometimes social workers disguise this basic reality in the pretense of professionalism. Another troublesome area associated with professionalism in advertising is the use of "professional jargon." Marketing plans in agencies today are seen as more professional, more objective and documented than in earlier days (Carson 1958: 170-171; Barton 1958:252-273). However, some of them are written in business lingo that are offensive rather than constructive and the vernacular would be preferred. To quote, "American businessmen are not taught that it is a sin to bore your fellow creatures" (Ogilvy 1963:71). Important to salesmanship is the process of re-selling the agency to clients. It is viewed as a never ending process and an important feature in the stability of agency—client relationships. According to Stebbins:

> The price of leadership is the price of place. You cannot expect to stand in the front *race* of your industry simply by right of conquest. You must either go on—or go back. (Stebbins 1957:159)

When a client hires the advertising agency it is because he has decided that it is the best available to him. Perhaps, social work services would be enhanced if clients had the option and the opportunity to "shop around" for the "best deal" in terms of services. This emphasis toward consumer orientation and consumer preference in providing service might well prove beneficial to social work.

There are many rules and guidelines for being a good client (Barton 1958:218-251; St. Thomas 1956:1-32; Groesbeck 1964:17-300). Of the many rules this writer selected two which seemed to him to be more applicable to social work. One dealt with emancipation and freedom. It is important that the agency be free from fear. Frightened people are powerless to produce good advertising. The preservation of the advertising agency's freedom is essential (Groesbeck 1964:37-40). A key element to this ideal relationship is permanency (Barton 1958:234-251). According to an expert in the field:

> . . . If permanency is to be achieved, it must be in the minds of the parties from the very beginning. It must be deliberately and consciously built into the relationship. (Ogilvy 1964:74)

Second, the selection process is vital. It is important to select the right agency (Groesbeck 1964:46-390; Barton 1958:234-257). This entails the process in which the client and agency are engaged in finding out and testing out the relationship. It is necessary to know if the agency people are liked. The relationship between client and agency has to be an intimate one and it becomes essential to have good relationships. For according to one author, "the chemistry of life has everything to do with the chemistry of sales" (Stebbins 1957:50).

IMPLICATIONS FOR SOCIAL WORK

What is a good advertisement? There seems to be three schools of thought. One school holds that a good advertisement is an advertisement with a client's O.K. on it. Another school accepts Raymond Rubicom's definition that an admirable piece of advertisement is one that is remembered for a long time by the public and the advertisement world. The third school holds that good advertisement is one which sells the product without drawing attention to itself. This school of thought rivets the subject's attention on the product. Instead of saying, "What a clever advertisement," the subject says, "I never knew that before. I must try that product." The customer has the impression that he has made his choice without help, guidance or suggestions from an advertisement (Ogilvy 1963:37-39). The ultimate to good advertising is advertising that convinces people that they are making free and independent choices (Freeman 1957:37). Perhaps it is this third school of thought that social workers have covertly practiced in their daily work activities. If this is the case, perhaps a more conscious and overt understanding and usage of this knowledge would enhance the social work professional. Perhaps it may be found that the ultimate to good advertising is as appropriate to social work as to advertising.

The question raised earlier in this paper dealt with the issue of the philosophical value base between the two fields of practice. The question posed pertained to whether there existed such an incompatability in the philosophical orientations of the two fields as to prohibit the utilization of knowledge between and within these two areas of practice. This writer contends the answer must be a strong *no!* This conviction has been reached after a careful review of the literature pertaining to the pros and cons of the merits of advertisement (Backman 1967; Barmin 1974; Lyon 1943; Barmash 1974; Stebbins 1957; Carson 1958: 20-223). This writer concurs with the writers who view good advertisement as fulfilling a social need and providing a useful and social function in society. This writer contends that the social work profession needs to become more responsive to and become cognizant of the knowledge and skills that can be learned and borrowed from advertising. The professional should be exposed to knowledge in advertising and salesmanship and social work education should be encouraged to expand its curriculum to include advertising in the training of social workers. This shift may necessitate a change in social work education and practice. This shift in orientation is addressed in Prigmore and Atherson. The authors discuss the outlook and future for social work. Their prospects for the future include a reorientation of social work values to reflect the values of society. They alert the social work profession to make better use of the existing values in society even though they may appear to be in conflict with social work values. An appeal is made for social workers to re-examine their position and to address practical concerns in the realm of social welfare policy. Their discussion on changes and innovations may appear formidable since they challenge the traditional model of practice and education. They foresee for the future the independent social work practitioner. Private practice is viewed as a healthy sign. Their vision includes a facility or firm consisting of specialists in specific problems that offer social work services at all levels from the individual to the community level. A firm of social work specialists who could and would contract planning services.

If this is any indication of the future, then it would appear most opportune for social workers to rethink and reshape their orientation to incorporate the advertising skills that would enhance their salesmanship. Prigmore and Atherson put forth a challenge to social workers. It is whether social workers can learn to become advocates, brokers, activists, and enablers with economic and educational institutions. They conclude by claiming why not, if social work skills are those of influencing, building, and utilizing relationships, perceiving interorganizational connections and fashioning new bridges (Prigmore and Atherson 1979: Chapter 8). The writer concludes this paper by extending this challenge to include salesmanship and advertising skills in their repertoire and ends with the words—"why not?"

BIBLIOGRAPHY

Backman, Jules; 1967-*Advertising and Competition.* New York: University Press.
Barmash, Isodora, 1974-*The World is Full of It.* New York: Delacorte Press.
Barron, Frank 1958-The Psychology of Imagination. *Scientific American.* 199 (3): 150-166.

Barton, Robert, 1958-*Advertising Agency Operations and Management.* (First Edition). New York: McGraw Hill Company, Inc.

Bedell, Clyde 1952-*How To Write Advertising That Sells.* New York: McGraw Hill Book Company, Inc.

Blumenthal, L. Roy 1972-*The Practice of Public Relations.* New York: The MacMillan Company.

Bronowski, J. 1958-The Creative Process. *Scientific American.* 199 (3): 59-65.

Cardamone, Tom 1959-*Advertising Agency and Studio Skills.* New York: Watson-Guptil Publications.

Carson, R. H. 1958-*Moguls of Merchandising...A History of The Carolinas.* Wilmington, N.C.: Jackson and Bell.

Clarke, R. N. 1978-Marketing Health Care: Problems in Implementation. *Health Care Management Review.* 3(1):21-27.

Freeman, William M. 1957-*The Big Name.* New York: Printers Ink Books.

Fryzel, R. J. 1978-Marketing Nonprofit Institutions. *Hospital and Health Services Administration.* 23(1):8-16.

Garton, T. 1978-Marketing Health Care: It's Untapped Potential. *Hospital Progress.* 59(2): 46-50.

Gottschall, Edward M. and Arthur Hawkins. 1959-*Advertising Directions.* New York: Art Directors Book Company.

Groesbeck, Kenneth 1964-*The Advertising Agency Business.* Chicago: Advertising Publications, Inc.

Kahn, Robert 1978-Prevention and Remedies. *Public Welfare.* 36(2):61-63.

Kotler, P. 1972-*Marketing Management: Analysis, Planning, and Control.* Englewood Cliffs, New Jersey: Prentice-Hall.

Kotler, P. and Zaltman, P. 1971-Social Marketing: An Approach To Planned Social Change. *Journal of Marketing Research.* 8(2):3-12.

Lovelock, C. H. 1977-Concepts and Strategies for Health Marketers. *Hospital and Health Services Administration.* 22(4):50-62.

Lyon, Margaurite 1943-*And So To Bedlam.* New York: The Bobbs-Merrill Company.

Maslach, Christina 1978-How To Cope. *Public Welfare.* 36(2):56-58.

McClure, Leslie W. 1950-*Newspaper Advertising and Promotions.* New York: The Mac-Millan Company.

McClure, Leslie and Paul C. Fulton 1964-*Advertising In The Printed Media.* New York: The MacMillan Company.

Ogilvy, David 1963-*Confessions Of An Advertising Man.* New York: Atheneum.

Prigmore, Charles S. and Charles R. Atherton 1979-*Social Welfare Policy: Analysis and Formulation.* Lexington, Mass.: D. C. Heath and Company.

Quelch, John A. 1980-Marketing Principles and the Future of Preventive Health Care. *Health and Society.* 58(2):310-347.

Rank, Otto 1958-*Beyond Psychology.* New York: Dover. 1968-*Will Therapy and Truth and Reality.* New York: Knopf Publishing Company.

Rapaport, Lydia 1968-Creativity in Social Work. *Smith College Studies in Social Work.* 38(3):139-161.

Rathmell, J. M. 1974-*Marketing and the Service Sector.* Cambridge, Mass.: Winthrop Publishers.

Rewoldt, S. H., Scott, J. D., and Warshaw, M. R. 1977-*Introduction to Marketing Management.* Homewood, Ill.: Richard D. Irwin.

Robinson, Virginia 1949-*The Dynamics of Supervision.* Philadelphia: The University of Pennsylvania Press.

Schwab, Victor O. 1962-*How To Write A Good Advertisement.* New York: Harper and Brothers Publishers.

Stebbins, Hal 1957-*Copy Capsules.* New York: McGraw-Hill Book Company, Inc.

St. Thomas, C. E. 1956-*How To Get Industrial and Business Publicity.* Philadelphia: Chilton Co.

PART IV:
SELECT RESEARCH CASES:
HOSPICE CARE, PARENTING,
AND DEINSTITUTIONALIZATION

Marketing can only be based on continued research which provides better insight into consumer and provider behavior. It is important to better understand the unique features of the services we are providing. These features provide a base from which to develop marketing strategies. In this section, the reader has three research projects related to hospice care, parenting and communication, and deinstitutionalization.

The first article on hospice care investigates the validity of marketing this type of service solely based on its cost-effectiveness over traditional in-patient care for terminally ill clients. This feature was a key reason why hospices were originally funded. It formed the framework for the majority of their marketing campaigns. The article definitely gives us new insight into this feature as well as reinforcing additional features which may be as effective in marketing hospice services.

The second article in this section also investigates features which differentiates parenting services. The emergence of numerous single parents, child abuse incidents, child care centers, family violence, and just general concern about parenting has been the stimulus for numerous parenting human and social services. Understanding the perceptions and characteristics of parenting and the interrelationship with communication techniques allows for improved service delivery and marketing success.

The third research area is applied to after-care for clients who have been in health institutions. A major problem area for successful services in this area is the lack of adequate living arrangements for these clients. In order to successfully market these

117

type of services to medical providers and the community it is important to understand how to communicate these needs. It also provides for a base of a new needed service in relation to finding living arrangements. There is a strong need to develop marketing programs related to marketing to discharge planners and people in the community who would be willing to provide these services.

There are many barriers to successfully marketing human and social services. Only through this kind of continued research will we be able to better serve our clients, as well as develop more effective communication and marketing programs. Effective communication is the base for successful marketing.

WJW

A Cost Analysis of Hospice Versus Non-Hospice Care: Positioning Characteristics for Marketing a Hospice

Kathleen Oji-McNair

INTRODUCTION

Health care costs in the United States have become a topic of increasing interest and controversy. In our struggle for stability, it would seem that healthcare is just another industry to be suffering under the economic pressure of the 1980's. However, healthcare in particular is undergoing intense scrutiny in terms of its rising costs. The statistics for calendar year 1978 for the United States was 192.4 billion for healthcare, accounting for 9.1% of the gross national product.[1] The situation continues to worsen as revealed in more recent statistics: "In 1981 American spent more than $278 billion on healthcare, nearly 10% of the gross national product."[2]

The consumer, provider, insurance and government are all in search of ways to curb these rising costs. With our aging population, Medicare in particular has become very conscious of being selective in what kinds of services it will reimburse.

One health service to recently come into use in the United States is hospice. It has been practiced in the Europe for many years and has come to describe institutions or programs designed to control and relieve the emotional and physical suffering of the terminally ill and to provide support for their families. It has received strong support and tremendous growth in its short life. In 1970, only 6 hospices were known to exist in the United States. By 1982, 440

Kathleen Oji-McNair, Health Consultant, Sacramento, California.

Special thanks to Dr. R. Goldman and Michael Tscheu who gave the primary guidance in the preliminary work of this study. Special acknowledgement and appreciation to the physicians, their staffs and the individuals in the institutions studied for their cooperation, assistance and support.

new hospices had been established with 350 in the planning stage.[3] Because nearly 60% of terminally ill cancer patients are over the age of 65, Medicare was very much interested in finding the most cost effective ways to care for these patients.[4] After studies on issues of cost effectiveness, the Federal government decided to increase Medicare reimbursement for hospice which has been available since November 1983. These pilot studies indicated substantial savings of hospice care versus non-hospice care. However, these studies mainly concentrated their savings claims on the number of inpatient days saved by the use of hospices. This study examines not only the number of inpatient days not utilized when hospice care is chosen, but it will determine what all the costs are for a sample of hospice patients versus a control group of inpatients who choose the traditional mode of care. Although reimbursement by Medicare has been hard fought for by hospices, it has become an area of much controversy as it imposes a cost cap considered by many to be insufficient and regulation that may cause hospice to reject this source of reimbursement.

METHODS

A. Subjects

This study was a retrospective, matched pair study. The subjects were stratified for sex, age and diagnosis. The cancer sites representing about 70% of all cancers for males and females for a three year period from a hospital based hospice program form the population. The ages were matched within 5 year intervals. From this population, 30 patients were chosen.

The control group represents 30 cancer patients who died and did not receive hospice services during the course of their illness. They were matched by age, sex and diagnosis to the hospice group. The population was limited to 6 physicians' practices. This was necessary to be able to determine the number of office visits, additional drug, equipment, etc., charges that were required when the patients were not in the hospital. These particular practices represented about 20% of all cancer admissions to the hospital for the time period between mid 1980 and mid 1983.

In order to determine how well the population studied represents other hospice programs, a survey of the population for 1980-1983 by diagnosis and sex was done. These two criteria were chosen as they are significant factors in determining the course of disease and therefore important factors in the type and extent of services utilized. A comparison with statistics from the American Cancer Society for 1982 can be seen in Table 1.

B. Research Design

The review period for each subject covered the last 55 days of life. This is the average number of days a patient is in a hospice program. The costs measured for the hospice population are as follows: (1) Number of days in the hospice program (includes administrative costs, overhead, hospital space for offices utilities, salaries); (2) number of visiting nurse visits; (3) inpatient and outpatient hospital costs; and (4) costs for radiation therapy, pharmacy consultation, social services, bereavement counseling and physician visits. The hospital population control group costs were established by review of patient charts, billing information, and physician records. This provided cost information for inpatient care, drugs, ancillary services, and physician charges (outpatient visits).

C. Procedure

Tables 2 and 3 represent the methodology used to determine the sample size for each site of disease so that the final sample would be representative of the total hospice population for mid 1980 to mid 1983. As shown, the disease sites for males and females representing approximately 70% of all sites for the hospice population are considered for the sample. Once these patients were selected the hospital's tumor registry was researched to identify patients who most closely match the hospice sample by age, sex and diagnosis. From that point, patients' charges, billing information, hospice data, etc., were accessed to determine what services were used and what costs were incurred for both populations.

RESULTS

The data gathered and compiled presents interesting findings which are dissimilar to previous studies on the cost savings of hospice. Table 4 is a summary comparing the costs of care of the 30 patients selected as representative of the total hospice population for

TABLE I

CANCER STATISTICS

Death by Site and Sex

MALE

American Cancer Society - U.S. 1982		Hospice Program 1981 - 1982
34%	Lung	43%
12%	Colon & Rectum	13%
10%	Prostate	8%
9%	Lymphomas	5%
65%		69%

FEMALE

American Cancer Society - U.S. 1982		Hospice Program 1981 - 1982
19%	Breast	24%
16%	Lung	22%
15%	Colon & Rectum	15%
5%	Ovary	7%
5%	Uterus	2%
5%	Pancreas	4%
65%		74%

TABLE 2

FEMALE HOSPICE PATIENTS
Calculations to Obtain Sample Size

SITE OF DISEASE	NUMBER PATIENTS	AVERAGE AGE	% OF TOTAL POPULATION ♀	6 SITES % OF TOTAL =	NUMBER OF PTS./SITE	NUMBER OF PTS. (rounded)
COLON & RECTUM	15	65	14%	18.3%	2.75	3
LUNG	26	64	25%	31.7%	4.76	5
BREAST	25	59	24%	30.8%	4.62	5
OVARY	7	59	6%	8.5%	1.28	1
UTERUS	5	70	4%	6.1%	.92	1
PANCREAS	4	75	3%	4.9%	.74	(1)*
	82 = 81% of total Hospice + 19 Other sites	65	76%	100%	15 ⟶	15 patients

Total ♀ pop. = 101

*This site was deleted as it represented the smallest percentage of the population (.74).

TABLE 3

MALE HOSPICE PATIENTS

Calculations to Obtain Sample Size

SITE OF DISEASE	NUMBER PATIENTS	AVERAGE AGE	% OF TOTAL ♂ POPULATION	6 SITES % OF TOTAL	NUMBER OF PTS./SITE	NUMBER OF PTS. (rounded)
PROSTATE	10	71	9%	13.0%	1.95	2
COLON & RECTUM	14	65	13%	18.2%	2.73	3
LUNG	48	66	43%	62.3%	9.35	9
LYMPHOMA	5	74	5%	6.5%	.98	1
	77	69	70%	100%	15.01 ⟶	15 patients

+ 34 other sites

Total ♂ pop. = 111

TABLE 4

COMPARISON OF COSTS OF CARE FOR 30 HOSPICE vs. 30 NON-HOSPICE PATIENTS

FOR THE LAST 55 DAYS OF LIFE

	# Inpatient Days	Costs of Inpt. Care	Physician Costs	Radiation Therapy	Home Health Services	Hospice	Total Average Cost/Patient
HOSPICE							
Total for each service	286	$125,785	$14,026	$10,174	$19,007	$42,324	
Average Cost per patient	9.53	$4193	$468	$339	$634	$1411	
Cumulative average cost of care/pt.		$4193	$4661	$5000	$5634	$7045	$7045
NON-HOSPICE							
Total for each service	437	$201,424	$15,069	$8944	$2243		
Average Cost per patient	14.37	$6714	$502	$298	$75		
Cumulative average cost of care/pt.		$6714	$7216	$7514	$7589	$7589	$7589
% Decreasing Savings for Hospice Patients with each additional service		38%	35%	33%	26%	7%	

the program evaluated over 3 years with the non-hospice control group of patients.

The bottom line of Table 4 indicates that after all the costs of hospice and non-hospice patients' care are totalled, the average savings per patient care in the last 55 days of life for hospice patients is 7%. The actual dollar difference represented by 7% is $544 per patient (or $7589 per non-hospice patient minus $544 per hospice patient average). This is substantially lower than any of the savings reported to date. Therefore, the findings affirm previous studies of hospice care saving costs but it is *very* qualified affirmation. As previously discussed, if only the number of inpatient days saved by use of hospice care are determined, the cost savings are substantial, representing a 38% saving. This statistic is consistent with many of the other studies and, in fact, correlates with the Blue Cross study finding of a cost saving of 39% for the last 8 weeks (56 days) of life.[5] It also compares with the findings of other studies that have looked at the comparative costs of care.[6,7,8,9] This study shows a cost per patient saving in hospital utilization alone to be $2521. The average reported saving for three of the studies previously sited is $2488. The difference being only $22.00 saved per hospice patients. However, as the other services are considered, the savings are not as dramatic.

The chart is designed to show the correlating decrease in the percent of cost savings as each service utilized by these patients are added. First, the physician costs for office and hospital visits, drug administration and purchase, etc., when added to the hospital utilization figure of percent savings (38%) lowers the difference to 35%. Next, costs for radiation therapy are added resulting in a decrease of relative savings to 33%. Home health services drop the difference to a 26% savings. Finally, a dramatic decrease of savings by hospice patients to 7% is observed when hospice costs are included.

A second consideration in this study was to look at the adequacy of the Medicare cap in relation to actual costs of hospice care. The final Medicare regulations stipulate a $6500 aggregate cap per patient. This means that for the hospice program considered in this study with an average cost per patient care of $7045, applying the Medicare cap of $6500, and with a population of 30 patients, the total costs not covered by Medicare would be $16,350 ($7045 minus $6500 = $445 × 30 = $16,350). The actual number of patients from the sample population was 212 over 3 years which would result in $115,540 not covered by Medicare for that time frame or $38,513 per year average. It should be noted that the reasons for the higher costs for radiation therapy in the hospice sample of 12% over the radiation therapy for the non-hospice sample is not clear. A comparison of radiation therapy for cancer patients in a larger population would need to be conducted to see if this holds true.

DISCUSSION

The results of this study are in agreement with previous investigations that, indeed, hospice care is less expensive than non-hospice care. However, the savings in this study have proven to be much less than previously reported. Some factors that may account for the difference in costs from other hospice programs studied could be: (1) costs of radiation therapy, physician office visits and procedures were not considered; (2) costs for the actual administration of the programs were not considered; and, (3) variance in the comprehensiveness of the program. These are only assumptions since there is no indication to the contrary for any of these studies. Taking only one of these factors into account, the costs of daily administration of such a program can drop the potential savings of hospice care almost 20%. Although it is difficult to say that this study is an actual comparison to other hospices surveyed because of these factors, the program studied has the outstanding results of its patients spending 90% of their days at home from the time they entered the program, an average saving of 5.4 hospital days per patient. This may be an indication that a comprehensive program such as the one studied may actually have a greater relative effectiveness in its allowing patients to remain at home with greater ease and confidence. A study to test the significance of the level of comprehensiveness of a hospice program to the relative costs may be of interest in determining if such a relationship exists.

An important area for consideration that has not been discussed in this study is the more difficult factors to measure such as success in pain control and patient/family satisfaction with the kind of care given when comparing hospice and traditional care. This has been the subject of another study by Kane et al. in which there was no difference in pain or symptom relief between the two types of care but that the patients and families in the hospice program studied expressed a greater degree of satisfaction with the kind of care they received.[10]

One might be tempted to conclude that since hospice care may not be as dramatic in its role of decreasing costs of care as previously reported, its value may be greatly minimized. This, however, has never been the main purpose of hospice care. It remains to be of significant value in the social and emotional aspects of the dying and their families and therefore should be encouraged to grow and become more available to those in need. Medicare reimbursement could be a vehicle to this end but may instead become a detriment to hospice programs by an insufficient cost cap and numerous regulations that may create more problems than help. It is for these reasons that a close accounting of costs of care on the part of hospices is necessary to determine their ability to operate and grow either with Medicare or without it.

It would seem that from whatever arena one is aligned with, i.e., third party payors, hospice service provider to hospital administration, careful investigation is to all parties' advantage to know as accurately as possible what the true costs are of hospice care and to consider the value of a comprehensive program.

FOOTNOTES

1. Charles H. White, PhD and Larkin E. Morse. *Hospital Fact Book.* Sacramento, California. Hospital Association. Sacramento: California Health Facilities Commission, November 1979.

2. The Sacramento Bee. "War on Medical Costs Creating Odd Bedfellows." March 1, 1982.

3. Michele L. Robinson. "Hospice Coverage Will Fuel Growth of Service" *Modern Health Care,* October 1982, p. 8.

4. Report to the Congress of the United States. "Hospice Care—A Growing Concept in the United States." United States General Accounting Office. March 6, 1979, p. 18.

5. Charles H. Brooks, PhD and Kathleen Smyth-Staruch, MA. Cost Savings of Hospice Home Care to Third-Party Insurers. Blue Cross of Northeast Ohio, September 1983, p. 14.

6. Anthony Amado, Beatrice A. Cronk, and Rich Mileo. "Cost of Terminal Care: Home Hospice vs. Hospital." *Nursing Outlook,* August 1979, pp. 522-526.

7. Linda Van Buren. "Hospice Home Care: A Cost Analysis of a Sample of Patients Seen During 1980". *Home Health Review,* September 1981.

8. Marie Kassakian, Linda R. Bailey, Marilyn Rinker, Carol Stewart, and Jerome W. Yates. "The Costs and Quality of Dying: A Comparison of Home and Hospital". *Nurse Practitioner,* January-February, 1979, pp. 18-23.

9. Bernard Bloom and Priscilla D. Kissick. "Home and Hospital Cost of Terminal Illness." *Medical Care,* May 1980, pp 560-564.

10. Robert Kane, Leslie Bernstein, Jeffrey Wales, Arleen Leibowitz and Stevan Kaplan. "A Randomised Controlled Trial of Hospice Care." *The Lancet,* April 21, 1984, p. 893.

BIBLIOGRAPHY

Amado, Anthony, Cronk, Beatrice A., and Mileo, Rich. "Cost of Terminal Care: Home Hospice vs. Hospital." *Nursing Outlook,* August 1979, pp. 522-526.

Bloom, Bernard S., and Kissick, Priscilla D. "Home and Hospital Cost of Terminal Illness." *Medical Care,* May 1980, pp. 560-564.

Brooks, Charles H., PhD and Smyth-Staruch, Kathleen, MA. Cost Savings of Hospice Care to Third Party Insurers. Blue Cross of Northeast Ohio, September 1983.

Kane, Robert L., Bernstein, Leslie, Wales, Jeffrey, Leibowitz, Arleen, Kaplan, Stevan. "A Randomized Controlled Trial of Hospice Care." *The Lancet,* April 21, 1984, pp. 890-894.

Kassakian, Marie, Bailey, Linda R., Rinker, Marilyn, Stewart, Carol A. and Yates, Jerome W. "The Costs and Quality of Dying: A Comparison of Home and Hospital". *Nurse Practitioner,* January-February, 1979, pp. 18-23.

Report to Congress of the United States. Hospice Care—A Growing Concept in the United States. United States General Accounting Office. March 6, 1979.

Robinson, Michele L. "Hospice Coverage Will Fuel Growth of Service". *Modern Health Care,* October 1982, p. 8.

The Sacramento Bee. "War on Medical Costs Creating Odd Bedfellows". March 1, 1982.

Van Buren, Linda. "Hospice Home Care: A Cost Analysis of a Sample of Patients Seen During 1980". *Home Health Review,* Sept. 1981.

White, Charles H. and Morse, Larkin E. *Hospital Fact Book.* Sacramento, California. Hospital Association, Sacramento: California Health Facilities Commission, November 1979.

Parenting and Communication: A Qualitative Analysis Key to Marketing Parenting Services

Jacques C. Bourgeois
Barbara Helm

INTRODUCTION

The Health Promotion Directorate of the federal department of Health and Welfare Canada has been investigating parents' perceptions of their information requirements with respect to child rearing. This research proposes to explore the nature of these information needs, which are presently believed to be primarily related to alcohol and drug issues. As well as these issues, other parental concerns are probed. Once the information needs are established, the means of delivering this information to parents is also investigated.

A companion paper addresses the parental concerns, roles, and knowledge levels. The present paper is directed at exploring information needs in terms of sources delivery systems, formats/media and type/content. This research is qualitative in nature and meant to serve as input to a national survey on parenting.

Jacques C. Bourgeois, President, DEMAND Research Consultants Inc., Division of Currie, Coopers & Lybrand, Ottawa, Ontario and Visiting Professor, Faculty of Administration, University of Ottawa.

Barbara Helm, Education Consultant, Health Promotion Directorate, Health and Welfare Canada, Ottawa, Ontario.

This research was supported in part by the Health Promotion Directorate, Health and Welfare Canada. Interpretations and recommendations expressed herein reflect the views of the authors and should not be interpreted as a statement of policy of Health and Welfare Canada.

LITERATURE REVIEW

Use of Mass Media

Advertising campaigns designed to mass market parenting concepts have been used by governments and have been fairly successful. The Ontario government test marketed their "You are not alone" advertisements with a 22% self-reported behaviour change. These TV advertisements were targeted to mothers of young children (under 5 years old) but mass marketed through commercial television (Ratcliffe and Wittman, 1983). The advertisements used an indirect approach. A group of Manitoba agencies is also intending to use a special cable programming channel during prime time to promote health and wellness.

Uses of Parenting Courses

Whether they are meant for general improvement of parenting skills or for coping with specific behaviour problems, most parenting courses are voluntary. Research has shown that the volunteers are those parents least in need of the parenting courses. They are well educated, have a higher than average socio-economic status and show great knowledge and concern about their child's behaviours. Because of the significantly different characteristics of these volunteers, the effectiveness of most voluntary parenting programs is limited. That is, these parents were found to have not significantly changed in knowledge, attitude, or behaviour (Albert and Simpson, in press). Stevens (1978) found that education and higher socio-economic status also determined whether the volunteer would show high involvement in the program. Anchor and Thomason (1975) sum up the volunteer phenomenon by saying that those who take parenting courses are the ones who need it least and the problem child is not reached in this way. Another problem associated with determining the effectiveness of parenting programs is the lack of a follow-up strategy (Whitehead and Gliksman, 1982).

Following are a few of the parenting courses either sponsored directly or indirectly by government. "STEP" (Systematic Training for Effective Parenting) uses an indirect approach to improve family relationships. It is assumed that everyone can improve. Leaders fairly rigidly adhere to the course outline which stresses that reward and punishment are counter productive. Another popular indirect approach program is "PET" (Parent Effectiveness Training). It is often used in conjunction with other more direct approaches to specific behaviour change (Rinn and Markle, 1977). When "PET" was compared to "Behaviour Modification Child Management Program", no difference was found and neither program showed any long term change (Albert and Simpson, in press).

Health-Risk Directed Programs

Programs have been developed to deal with specific health-risk behaviours in mind. Drug abuse is indirectly approached using "Creating Supportive Systems". This program approaches, in a direct manner, the skills for creating cohesive family interactions. Whitehead and Gliksman (1982) state that there is no support for an indirect approach to drug abuse without, as well, some sort of direct approach. "Kids and Drugs" is another indirect approach. It is based on the "STEP" parenting program.

The indirect approach is also being used in the prevention of alcohol abuse. One of the programs (i.e., "All in the Family") uses awareness as its target of change. There is little support for this approach since direct knowledge is said not to affect appropriate alcohol-related behaviour. A similar program, "Decisions in Drinking" was carried out in Ontario with very poor results. The parents (of children less than 10) were so removed from any perceived risk that there was no change. They actually left feeling less concerned than before the course (Albert, Simpson and Eaglesham, 1982). This program was also used in the United States ("Power of Positive Parenting") but is no longer being reprinted. The Canadian government is sponsoring an alcohol abuse prevention program ("Dialogue on Drinking") which uses an indirect and direct approach using information, awareness and action as its focus.

Bukoski (1982) sums up his review of prevention programs by stating that there is no drug abuse prevention program which has been successful. However, one program that has been successful is the saying "no" strategy for cigarette smoking. By using positive peer pressure techniques, there has been a 50% reduction in onset. This effect has also been carried over into other related behaviours of alcohol, and marijuana.

METHODOLOGY

Market Coverage

The focus group composition was meant to reflect a representation of population density, region, language, sex, and S.E.S. (see Exhibit 1). Thirteen focus groups and 13 depth interviews were conducted across Canada during the month of January (1983).

Participant Characteristics

The participants to all focus groups and depth interviews were parents of children between the ages of 5 and 14 (with a recruiting emphasis on 8-11 year olds), living with their children. The par-

EXHIBIT I

POPULATION CHARACTERISTICS 1
OF
FOCUS GROUP SITES

	Population	Family Size	% Own
Atlantic			
Amherst N.S.	10,260	3.3	64%
Moncton (Metro), N.B.	77,570	3.5	61
Quebec			
Plessisville	7,240	3.5	65%
Victoriaville	27,730	3.5	60
Quebec (Metro)	542,160	3.5	46
Ontario			
Stratford	25,655	3.3	66%
Toronto (Metro)	2,803,100	3.3	56
Prairies			
Indian Head, Sask.	1,720	3.0	81%
Regina (Metro) Sask.	151,190	3.4	65
B.C.			
Hope	2,960	3.3	66%
Port Coquitlam	23,930	3.5	82
Vancouver (Metro)	1,166,350	3.2	59
CANADA	**22,992,600**	**3.5**	**63%**

---

1   Data obtained from 1976 Census - Statistics Canada

ticipants were selected from each appropriate area telephone directory and/or through a referral system. The demographic characteristics of the 84 focus group participants are detailed in Exhibit 2 by region and in total. In addition, participants had to:

   i. meet all the specified screening criteria (i.e., sex, marital status S.E.S. age and language)
   ii. not have attended a focus group in the past 12 months
   iii. not have attended a focus group on child rearing in the past 24 months and,
   iv. not work for a market research company, a department of Health and Welfare (federal or provincial) or in a position dealing with child rearing (e.g., psychologist counsellor).

Procedure

Following an introduction, the discussion developed in a "funnel approach". That is the discussion began with a general talk of their thoughts about their children and child rearing, then, about concerns they may have with respect to their children; followed by a more specific discussion on the types of information sought and/or previously obtained and their sources.

Along with this discussion, participants were asked to express their opinions in writing to questions on each of several potential parental concerns. This was followed, in each case, by a discussion of the particular parental concern most important to them.

INFORMATION SOURCES

Basic Findings

Nine basic information sources were identified through the focus groups. Those of prime importance were (in decreasing order of importance): friends/family/relatives, school/teachers/counsellors, professional, church, and government departments or service branches. Those of a secondary importance were identified as: library, instinct/commonsense/experience, non-profit organizations, and other organisms (e.g., police, private sector and drugstore). Importance is judged here by the participants' stated preference for one source vs another.

Although this second group of information sources were labelled

EXHIBIT 2

DEMOGRAPHIC COMPOSITION
OF
FOCUS GROUP PARTICIPANTS

CHARACTERISTICS	REGION					TOTAL	
	ATLANTIC	QUEBEC	ONTARIO	PRAIRIES	B.C.	N	%
SEX:							
male	9	3	10	4	10	36	43
female	9	9	10	11	11	48	57
MARITAL STATUS:							
married	13	6	14	7	20	60	72
separated/divorced							
widowed	5	6	4	7	1	23	28
OCCUPATION:							
professional/managerial	2	2	8	1	3	16	19
sales	2	–	1	–	2	5	6
clerical	1	2	2	2	2	9	11
skilled labour	2	–	1	3	3	9	11
unskilled labour	3	2	3	4	2	14	17
housewife	8	5	2	4	8	27	32
unemployed	–	1	1	1	–	3	4
OCCUPATION OF SPOUSE:							
professional	2	2	3	–	–	7	12
managerial	1	–	1	–	–	2	3
sales	–	–	–	–	1	1	2
clerical	3	–	2	1	1	7	12
skilled labour	2	3	1	2	5	13	22
unskilled labour	2	–	–	4	5	11	19
housewife	3	–	7	–	8	18	30
unemployed	–	1	–	–	–	1	2
HOUSEHOLD INCOME:							
less than $10,000	5	1	–	5	1	12	14
$10,001 to $15,000	2	2	2	6	3	15	18
$15,001 to $20,000	4	3	5	2	2	16	20
more than $20,000	6	6	11	2	14	39	48
average ($)	17,833	22,100	23,592	13,713	24,600	20,746	
CHILDREN AGED:							
less than 5	4	2	7	7	12	32	15
5, 6 or 7	6	5	8	11	10	40	18
8 to 11	15	10	16	16	17	74	34
12 13 or 14	6	6	7	7	12	38	17
15 or 16	6	1	5	2	7	21	10
more than 16	6	1	–	–	5	12	6
average (years)	9.6	6.4	9.5	8.7	9.2	9.3	
NO. OF CHILDREN:							
1	4	3	3	1	–	11	13
2	7	6	8	5	10	36	43
3	3	2	4	5	7	21	25
4 or more	4	1	3	4	4	16	19
average	2.4	1.4	2.3	2.8	3.1	2.5	
LANGUAGE:							
French	6	12	0	0	0	18	21
English	12	0	18	15	21	66	79
NUMBER OF GROUPS	3	2	3	2	3	13	

as being of secondary importance, they were perceived nonetheless as being quite important (not including the "other" category).

Language Differences

The French participants only distinguished themselves along one information source. That is, they were more likely to have used a government department or one of its service branches. Both language groups would not seem to differ in the importance they attach to two other sources of information (i.e., friends/family/etc., and library).

The English language group disproportionately prefers schools and their staff, professionals, Church, common sense/experience, and non-profit organizations (e.g., the Simon Fraser health clinic).

Community Size Differences

All three community sizes are similar in their relative preference for friends/etc., and Church. Rural participants favour government departments, schools and their staffs, and professionals. The participants from small-urban areas favor, as do the rural people, professionals. The large-urban participants tended to have a greater cross-section of information sources, including schools, libraries, common sense and N.P.O's.

Socio-Economic Status Differences

The lower and the middle/upper S.E.S. groups were relatively similar in four of their information sources (i.e., friends, school, government departments, and libraries). In only two cases are they different. The lower S.E.S. is less likely to contemplate using professionals and a Church.

Sex Differences

Females look more favorably on a Church as a source of information while males are relatively more likely to revert to their common sense/instinct and libraries. In a group discussion, females were also more likely to have stated a preferred use of government departments and professionals. At the females' suggestions, males also agree to the use of these sources.

INFORMATION MEDIUM/FORMAT

Basic Findings

There would seem to be no consensus on the preferred format for disseminating the information. Although, there are two generally more acceptable formats (i.e., books and TV). Following these two formats are eight other formats. In decreasing order of preference, these are: newspapers, magazines, pamphlets, meetings/group discussions/panels, films/documentaries, courses/lectures, word-of-mouth. Basically, those who sought information from a book desired a bit more depth information, in addition to having the flexibility of absorbing the information at their own pace and time. On the other hand, a significant number of participants would not really put out an effort to acquire the information. Therefore, TV (as a passive medium) would fulfill their needs.

Language Differences

English participants considered significantly more types of formats. Six formats (i.e., books, newspapers, word-of-mouth, meetings, magazines and films/documentaries) were significantly more preferred by the English Canadian participants. TV, pamphlets and courses/lectures were not relatively preferred by either group.

Community Size Differences

Rural communities would rather receive the information through TV and courses/lectures. Large-urban communities have a relative preference for books and newspapers. The small-urban communities have no strong preference, except perhaps for some inclination towards magazines.

Socio-Economic Status Differences

In two cases (newspapers and group meetings) both S.E.S. have relatively similar format preferences. Although, they do differ. The middle/upper S.E.S. group would relatively prefer magazines while the lower S.E.S. group attaches much greater importance to books, TV and pamphlets.

Sex Differences

The group conversations yielded differences in the sex of the participant. Males were much more likely to prefer books, TV, newspapers and word-of-mouth. Females would side with pamphlets and group meetings. No sex differences were observed for TV as a potential medium.

INFORMATION TYPE

Basic Findings

The type of information reported as being most sought is information related to drugs. As mentioned earlier, participants felt very ignorant about drugs. They not only feel a knowledge void about drugs, but they would also like this void filled.

There are two other areas where information is primarily sought: sexual behaviour, child development, and child rearing practices. Child development basically includes information sought on the various stages which a child experiences. Other types of information were also mentioned but were attributed less importance, these are: education, nutrition, communication, alcohol, and general health and welfare.

Language Differences

The need for information on drugs and on child development was relatively similar across both language groups. The French Canadian participants, on the one hand, were more likely to have sought information regarding "sexual behaviour" while on the other hand, the English participant has a broader repertoire of sought information. They had sought information on child rearing practices, education, nutrition and communication. Communication is defined as information which was sought to help the child and parent better communicate.

Community Size Differences

All three community sizes similarly sought information on drugs and sexual behaviour, though differences in other types of sought information do exist. For instance, the rural participants had the greatest information needs. They sought information with respect to child development, communication, child rearing practices and education.

The small-urban centers expressed a preference for information on alcohol and nutrition. The large-urban participants were relatively more likely to voice having sought information on child development.

Socio-Economic Status Differences

Differences were as well observed here. The middle/upper S.E.S. group of participants voiced a relatively stronger need for information on sexual behaviour. The lower S.E.S. group was more likely to have sought out information on child development, child rearing practices, education and parent-child communication. These two groups were not differentially likely to have sought out information on drugs.

Sex Differences

"All male" groups tended relatively to focus on child rearing practices as a sought type of information. On the other hand, "all female" groups were more likely to concentrate on parent-child communication and on child development. Similarly, the "mixed" group reported having sought information on drugs and child development. In addition, three other areas of sought information emerged: nutrition, child rearing practices and general health and welfare.

EMERGING ISSUES

Throughout the focus groups, several issues were discussed some more tangential than others. The major findings were reported earlier, following is a list of other emerging issues:

1. The participants usually reacted favorably to the fact that the Federal Department of Health & Welfare was the sponsor;
2. Rural participants were more open and honest. Their answers seemed less affected by the presence of other participants around the table.
3. A group discussion with participants who know each other in a

rural area does not seem to affect their opinions as much as those who know each other in a more urban center.

4. TV was very often pointed to as the culprit for supplying too much and/or the wrong information.

5. Of great importance to this study, is the fact that parents of children between the ages of 7 to 12 do not generally require information because they typically perceive themselves as not facing any serious problem during this stage. Thus, they reason that without a problem, there is no need for the information. They do not plan ahead, but rather react to a situation/problem. They are not concerned about a potential problem unless there is a problem.

6. Parents seek and extract only that parental information which is concordant with their beliefs about the particular situation at hand. In other words, they believe that there's their way and there's the wrong way!

7. Teachers are perceived as a good source to tell you the status of your child and those in the same stage as he/she is. But a teacher is not perceived as necessarily the proper source for advice re—a particular problem.

CONCLUSIONS AND RECOMMENDATIONS

Conclusions

From the preceding findings the following conclusions were drawn:

i. Parents of children aged 5 to 14, and especially 8-11, do not generally perceive any child rearing problem with their children (of this age). Since they *do not perceive a problem,* they as well *do not perceive a need for information* on child rearing for children of this age group.

ii. Unless there is a perceived need for information, *communication efforts* are *likely* to be very *ineffective.*

iii. The more important *information sources* were (in decreasing order of importance): friends/family/relatives, school/teachers/counsellors, professionals, Church, and government departments.

iv. The two most acceptable *information formats* are books and

TV. Others were also uncovered (in decreasing order of importance): newspaper, magazines pamphlets, meetings/ groups/discussions/panels, films/documentaries, courses/ lectures, and word-of-mouth.

v. Participants' reactions suggest that the audience is receptive to a *Federal promotional effort.*

vi. *Pamphlets* are not perceived as a medium with much depth of information.

vii. The most sought *information type* is drugs, followed closely with sexual behaviour, child develoment, and child rearing practices. Other information types, although of lesser importance were: education, nutrition, communication, alcohol, and general health and welfare.

viii. Differences and similarities in demographics and S.E.S. were uncovered for the different information sources, formats, and types.

Policy Recommendations

i. Communication efforts should be targeted to the various *"concern segments"*. Each segment should have a distinct message and appeal.

ii. *Pamphlets* should be intended to create awareness, and not depth of knowledge.

iii. The *promotional campaign* should follow a staged approach. Starting with specific campaigns, in the *short run* (i.e., 1-2 years) oriented at raising the target audience's awareness to relevant concerns. The campaign should then direct itself, over the *longer run* (i.e., 5-8 years), at changing behaviours. In the *medium turn,* changing attitudes towards the target concerns would likely improve the probability of changing behaviours in the long run.

iv. *Information sessions* (à la Tupperware) should be used as a communication means.

v. A more formalized *information network* should be set-up with the relevant professionals.

vi. The Department should *significantly* increase the awareness of the available information within Health and Welfare Canada.

vii. More stress should be put on the development of *booklets* presenting detailed information organized by concern area.

viii. A weekly *newspaper column* should be organized.

BIBLIOGRAPHY

Albert, N.G. & R.L. Simpson (in press), "Test Construction Procedures for the Evaluation of Alcohol Education", *International Journal of the Addictions.*

Albert, W.G., R.L. Simpson, and J.A. Eaglesham (1982), "Evaluation of a Drinking and Parenting Educational Programme in Six Ontario Communities" (Sept.).

Anchor, K.N. and T.C. Thomason (1975), "A Comparison of Two-Parent-Training Models with Educated Parents", *Journal of Community Psychology* 5, 134-141.

Bukoski, W.J. (1982), "Drug Abuse Prevention Research: An Outline for Action" Health Promotion/Disease Prevention Research Seminar, Montreal, Nov. 11-12.

Rinn, R.C. and Markle, A. (1977), "Parent Effectiveness Training, A Review", *Psychological Reports* 4, 95-109.

Ministry of Health, Ontario (1982), "Just Ask Us", Government of Ontario, Queen's Park, Toronto.

Ratcliffe, W.D. & Wittman, W.P. (1983), "Parenting Education: Test-Market Evaluation of a Media Campaign", *Prevention In Human Services* (Spring).

Stevens Jr., J.H. (1978), "Parent Education Programs: What Determines Effectiveness?" *Young Children* (May) 59-65.

Whitehead, P.C. & Gliksman, L. (1982), "Parenting Programs: A Review and Analysis" Prepared for H.P.D. (Dec).

A Systems Design Developmental Model for Programs of Deinstitutionalization: Marketing Base for Follow-Up Care

Salvatore Imbrogno

ABSTRACT. Devising plans to maintain individuals with a chronic mental disability in the community following a long-term hospitalization is a highly complex problem. One of the significant aspects of this problem is the availability of adequate living arrangements that promote individual growth and development, provide professional support and care, and elicit the concern of members in the community who will provide these living arrangements.

Alternate living arrangements require social experimentation in efforts to ascertain and appraise which one(s) are most appropriate for any given community. This paper devises a method of sequential development of alternatives in which each arrangement is appraised as it emerges in the community in relation to cost, knowledge acquired and utilized, technology advanced, and other resources required. It was assumed that each living arrangement produces different results in development. It further assumes that each living arrangement learns in development to the best interest of the chronic mentally disabled. The result of this innovative systems design is that professionals can make decisions on placement based on knowledge, information, technology, and cost as it emerges in juxtaposition to the results such programs are having on those in need.

I. INTRODUCTION

A novel way for planning comprehensive community based programs for patients re-entering the community is through the creation and implementation of a systems design development model. A systems design refers to a program planning process of arranging and rearranging the human, social and technical resources necessary to realize the desired results of deinstitutionalization. Intrinsic to a systems design conceptualization is the notion that social change occurs

---

Salvatore Imbrogno, Professor at the Ohio State University College of Social Work, 1947 College Road, Columbus, OH.

in turbulence in which the interactive processes of the program design are effected by and in turn effect the external environmental conditions in which it evolves.[1]

A systems design development model is programed to do a great deal of learning from experience as it is continuously confronting and solving problems in development. This requires a self-renewal phenomenon in the form of acquiring and utilizing new knowledge, technology and information. The learning and problem solving process enables the systems designer to change plans and directions as the program progresses sequentially through its various stages of development.

This paper will examine the conceptual foundation to a systems design model by describing the following stages of development for the formulation and implementation of a program of deinstitutionalization:

1. *Program planning*: comprises a comprehensive systematic study of the deinstitutionalization of the chronically mentally ill, projects explored as appropriate for re-entry into the community and the resources needed and available in the community for its realization.

2. *Exploratory project planning*: includes problem formulation in specificity; objectives to be selected in a search for or in pursuit of the policy goals; that a systems synthesis take place for compiling and/or inventing alternative living arrangements; that systems analysis follow in which the consequences and/or effects of each alternative be deduced; and finally, that the best systems for the social design operation be selected.

3. *Developmental project planning*: involves making necessary modifications and changes in all aspects of the system design if and when more efficient and effective ways are found to meet the multiplicity of needs of the chronically mentally ill.

4. *Community developmental planning*: entails a critical role for the community as a participatory and complementary support system in all stages of the system design development. The community in the last analysis determines through a variety of feedback processes if the system design is functioning satisfactorily.

This conceptual scheme is presented in a logical sequence of development. It is not, however, a linear causal model that has a beginning and end with no mutual interaction processes between each stage. Each stage can take the initiative to produce changes as the model evolves in development. In this regard, the effects of any one stage effects all others equally in that they are interconnected and interrelated. A systems design model is multicausal primarily intent on producing desired results in multifinality.[2]

II. PROGRAM PLANNING
IN A COMPREHENSIVE SYSTEM STUDY

Deinstitutionalization is a consequence of a social policy which authorizes decisions in program planning as steps toward policy implementation. There is no formalized or universally accepted strategy to follow in determining what a comprehensive delivery system entails nor is there general agreement as to how best to effectuate a program once it has been decided upon. Deinstitutionalization perceived from a systems construct, involves a program of strategies and tactics as the means for tackling an original problem in social planning for the chronically mentally ill. The reasons for viewing deinstitutionalization as an original problem are disclosed in the expectations intrinsic to these policies:

1. communities must realize that the chronically mentally ill are individuals who have different needs for services and that, in fact, these individuals have a multiplicity of complex needs of a chronic nature requiring long-term care;
2. the multiplicity and diversity of individual needs present a formidable task in the assignment of alternative living arrangements in the community, requiring a broad base complementary support system to provide appropriate long-term care and treatment;
3. the ultimate goal of a program of deinstitutionalization is the acceptance of the chronically mentally ill as full members of the community which requires that the complex network of services for them be an integral part of the community at large.

A fundamental requirement is to design a system capable of achieving policy goals under changing conditions through a program planning process of rational and creative action. This process must be so designed to acquire and utilize emerging knowledge, experience as it accumulates, and information necessary to establish the feasibilities of what is needed and to determine how best to actualize these needs. A planning problem to achieve a specific objective in a single living arrangement for one patient is different from problems where the objective(s) are to provide a comprehensive delivery system that meets the multiple and complex needs of a chronically mentally ill patient in a community over a long period. These conditions for program planning serve as the referents for other stages of development.

Hence, the initial purpose for program planning is to conduct a system study to achieve the following:

1. The first aim is to assist all those involved in the program to reach agreements on the total program planning and project objectives of the systems design.
2. This involves specifying the alternative living arrangements; the total community resources available and to be distributed to the various projects.
3. Most critical to a systems study is to create an extensive background of information on which to subsequently build in the planning of specific projects so that a proper approach of breadth and scope can be initiated and available to impending changes.

Program planning methods are used for planning strategies of involving patients, professionals and complementary specializations in group decision making processes:

1. coordinate the best use of experts in mental health decision making, patients, and citizens in the planning process;
2. plan programs involving different complementary specializations, such as health, rehabilitation, educational planning, etc.;
3. develop consensus in group decision making when participants from widely different backgrounds are involved;
4. legitimate decisions in the minds of the community in order to increase public acceptance of programs.[3]

This program planning method is purposefully designed to achieve desired results: (1) innovative and effective systems are to be designed rather than patched up versions of existing systems or solutions; (2) these designed systems have a plan for implementation; (3) a conceptual framework exists by placing emphasis on a desired system rather than an improvement of current community systems; (4) generate alternative solutions to a problem and (5) develop new community resources and services.

Techniques for generating ideas and gathering information in the community are brainstorming, synectics and delphi and for highly structured group interacting processes, nominal group processes. For the prescriptions in a systems design, "ideals strategy" is still another technique that can be presented to the community by the designer.

III. EXPLORATORY PROJECT PLANNING

The following living arrangements have been studied and are ready to be explored in development: (1) adoption as an alternative to residential services; (2) surrogate parents as substitutes for children's residential services; (3) natural homes for the institutionalized patient; (4) personal assistance as a basis for community living for adults; (5) community group homes as an alternative to institutionalized services; (6) apartment clusters in semi-independent living arrangements.[4] Let us assume that alternative living arrangements have been formalized in a systems study and are now ready to enter a project planning stage. The project planning stage in contemplating these alternatives requires decisions on what comprises a comprehensive delivery system for deinstitutionalization. Can it be integrated within a given community; can it be quantified relative to a community structure; can its patients and support systems be identified and defined within these project parameters?

In essence, there exist an array of living arrangements not all of which have transferable value to all communities. Some of these living arrangements take on a different structure and purpose when they are adapted by another community; others are integrated to form different configurations; all of which in a circular interaction with one another produce in totality a comprehensive system for a community that is quite different from each living arrangement taken separately.

A. Selecting Objectives

Project planning must resolve a major problem of interconnecting the goal of a comprehensive delivery system with the objectives of a systems design. The objectives now require more specificity than what was the case under goal formulation during system studies. For example, the strategic planning objectives require logistic "know what and know how" in the organization and management of the systems design relative to existing and emerging community resources as a complement to the "know where" of goal formulation in program planning.

Hence, in the early stages of exploratory project planning a major task is to acquire and utilize appropriate technology techniques necessary to actualize the systems design objectives. The objectives specified in turn, serve as guides in the search for alternatives, their feasibilities and actualization; objectives suggest the type of analysis required for studying alternatives and they provide criteria for selecting the best possible arrangements for the patient. Defining objectives is a universal imperative of a systems approach. There are techniques that focus on structuring objectives on hierarchical levels (objective trees and intent structures). A systems functional perspective on objectives can be realized in "functional expansion" techniques.

B. Systems Synthesis and Systems Analysis

Complex human and social needs of the chronically mentally ill can only be met by a multipurpose, well differentiated and highly consolidated and centralized system which must include a multiple combination of alternative living arrangements. This program and its project, therefore, becomes a system with a collection of function and processes which are interacting to achieve the purpose of deinstitutionalization. Identifying the salient interactions and describing their relationships is a very necessary next step to a social design model in development.

As noted, a comprehensive delivery system is a collection of alternative living arrangements which interacts to achieve specific functions and purposes (desired results). This notion permits the designer to describe the problem and prescribe a solution. A system definition matrix is a prescriptive technique for a systems analysis of the conditions and details that need to be specified in developing a social design. It also serves as a descriptive technique for understanding and specifying the multiple interactions and interrelations of the social design function and its internal environment. It imposes a morphological structure on a conceptual systems design model to produce prescriptions and descriptions of the functions and processes. A system definition matrix provides a checklist to guide information gathering for analysis as well as a format for specifying details of the social design. Describing complex relationships in systems synthesis requires sets of techniques that can identify and define the interactions in hierarchical relationships (i.e., tree diagraming): cross interactional relationships (matrix diagrams) and in feedback relationships (oval diagraming).[5]

C. Cost/Benefit Analytical Techniques

One of the major barriers to initiate, maintain, and sustain a system design for deinstitutionalization is funding. Under current reimbursement policies it is difficult to develop sufficient funding patterns that will encourage a program with a wide range of alternative living arrangements. A problem exists too in support of ongoing training, on-the-job training and where needed, support from community agencies over the long run. Public agencies do enter into a separate contract with the participants of the program for:

a. specific complementary specializations help in working with the chronically mentally ill, such as assistance in specific daily living skills, or meeting medical transportation needs;
b. for the provision in training of complementary specializations; and back up teams for coverage and to enhance overall capability; and to stabilize the turnover in support system.

The existing funding patterns in a community for support are critical to this system. However, most critical are the methods and techniques for financial control and accountability. That guarantees this system's viability and credibility.

A major technique advanced in mental health is the weighting of project benefits against the cost (cost/benefit analysis). In an emerging design, the time stream of benefits and costs must also be considered (cash/flow analysis) in order to analyze the design's alternatives in development. It is anticipated that changes in cost will occur in progress so that discounting technique provides a basis for analyzing and comparing future streams of cost and benefits by reducing them to their equivalent present worth. Various techniques are available to decide on the merits of alternative living arrangements, as for example net present worth, benefit cost ratio and internal rate of return.[6]

This exploratory project planning stage must be approached in terms of the complex relations in which learning about new methods and techniques for solving problems will take place. An analysis and synthesis occurs throughout the design process and not necessarily in chronological order. The systems design may be confronted with serious technical problems very late in development. This may occur because in the initial stages of the systems design these problems were not anticipated or the design was not conducted to uncover them. Or it may be, because some of the later "cost/benefit" ratio turn out to be so serious that it becomes necessary to change living arrangements. This in turn gives rise to a new series of technical problems. It is this stage of exploratory development however, that defines problems, selects objectives, is involved in systems synthesis and analysis in which the best system is selected for the patient.

IV. DEVELOPMENTAL PROJECT PLANNING

Experiences with systems design models in development indicate that one of the most unpredictable things about any new approach is how reliable will be the performance of the model. One of the main reasons why developmental costs and technological requirements are so seriously underestimated, is that tendency to minimize the problems in performance reliability that will be encountered and the amount of testing and modification that will be necessary to overcome them. For example, one of the most formidable problems in deinstitutionalization is making reliable case assignments based on the patient's "diagnosis" relative to the appropriate living arrangement. As with earlier stages of development these problems will have been anticipated to some degree in the initial stages of the systems design formulation. However for these problems to be systematically studied in detail, development of this systems design must progress to a point where a good deal is known and experienced about chronically mentally ill patients (i.e., the kinds of living arrangements that are feasible and desirable to the individual.)[7]

A. Action Phase in Project Planning

Each living arrangement becomes a discrete but coherent part of the whole comprehensive system design. In other words, each living arrangement has a clearly defined purpose which is congruent with the needs of the people in need of that service. Further, each must be clearly differentiated in its function, in its time of day, in its location, and in its staff identity so that patient needs are successfully met.

A series of questions might be asked of any living arrangement: are the right people (staff) serving the right people (patients), grouped in the right ways, doing things, and using the right methods? And are they doing it consistently and coherently? These are tactical questions to ensure efficient operations. Remember that strategic questions were responded to in exploratory project planning (i.e., relations between and within living arrangements).

Whether each living arrangement is viewed as a system or subsystem, a critical path method can build in logical and rational controls for project planning. A CPM can also be used as an aid in managing case assignments where activities must be performed in a specified sequence. This method can increase the rate and efficiency of placements that can be made by systematizing service developmental activities in planning chart which demonstrates the sequence of interdependencies of activities. *Gantt Charts* is a complementary technique that can be used to determine the project's activities given that resources are limited or even unavailable.[8]

B. Studies in Development

A major aim of a system design developmental model is to anticipate the changing needs and requirements of the chronically mentally ill in development. Patients as they become active members of the community are expected to progress let us say, from a highly structured setting where they are grouped together and share similar needs to a more independent, less structured environment. Other chronically mentally ill might regress in their assigned living arrangement. Careful observation and measurement of adjustments and changes must be conducted for every individual case. This suggests that research and evaluation of individual physiological and psychological functioning is a critical component to a system design model.[9] This becomes the role and function of the complementary support system and the designs information reporting system that ensures that this information is available to the system.

However, there are a number of problems that cannot be anticipated and arise only in development as the patient, living arrangements and community support systems converge to meet the multiplicity of complex needs and requirements. A systems design to work effectively and efficiently must therefore be redesigned as these new patterns and relations evolve. As noted, a model in development is a learning system that acquires and utilizes new knowledge, information and experience at its various stages in development. New patterns and relations will emerge in development and in so doing, change the direction of its plans and purpose. It is possible too, that failure of efforts to solve problems within existing plans, leads to shifts in the design assumptions about the patient and system—a change in the designer's understanding of the social reality relative to the patient and community support system.

For example, experience has shown that what was assumed to be taken as a need for residential service was different from how others perceived it. For example, a family's request for residential placement might arise from any one or a combination of need.

a. individual need, for instance for frequent medical services, assistance in achieving mobility or assistance in changing disruptive behavior;
b. family need, for example, arising from marital discord, inability of a caretaking person to continue to provide for the person, or uncertainty regarding their long-term ability to provide;
c. community related needs such as the lack of locally available resources or local intolerance of some conditions of behavior.

This more complex awareness of the nature of the chronically mentally ill patients needs, leads to different operations for service delivery. The chances of a system design model to operate reliably depends as much on trial and error as it does on the personal experiences and ingenuity of professionals and complementary specializations involved in operations as for example: (1) material supports, i.e., provisions for prosthetic and medical equipment; (2) removal or architectural barriers to mobility; and (3) provisions for time saving appliances such as washing machines and access to public transportation.

Successful implementation and management of a comprehensive and complex systems design depends largely on careful attention to detail. As noted, diagramming the sequence of necessary activities (critical Path method) and scheduling according to available resources (Gantt charts) assist this process. All these techniques ensure reliability of a systems design by stressing systematic analysis under changing conditions with emphasis on results. Most importantly, a systems design in development must possess in its format the capacity to change an initial design, its functional plans to meet internal and external changing conditions as they evolve in progress. This is a critical cybernetic process to the action phase of planning deinstitutionalization programs.

V. COMMUNITY DEVELOPMENTAL PLANNING

The final stage involves ascertaining and appraising if this system design is operating satisfactorily in the community. The actual environment under which a new program will be operationalized can be found to be quite different from the assumed conditions. For example, it might be falsely assumed that every community will resist efforts to have the chronically mentally ill in their midst or that every chronically mentally ill patient has a family (or relatives) that are able and willing to assume responsibility even with substantial, easily accessible support systems. A widely held belief is that the chronically disabled child is not adoptable and as a result, limited organized activities exist to seek adoptive homes. Experience has shown that when these assumptions are challenged and systematic approaches are introduced to search for homes and communities are engaged, support is gained for the program.

Traditionally, the preparation to move a chronically mentally ill patient out of an institution was done by the professional and patient just prior to deinstitutionalization. Experience here too shows that the patient's movement in a community placement is more contingent on the degree to which the community and its support systems are prepared for the patient than how the patient is made "readied" for the community. The natural or surrogate living arrangement it was argued must be prepared emotionally, intellectually and behaviorally to accept the patient and where the patient is.[10]

The community and its citizenry will be better able to respond positively to the needs and requirements of the chronically mentally ill when they are involved in all stages of the systems design's developmental process. The community must be offered an acceptable and understandable role to fulfill and an adequate support system to do so. The community and its members in the program must be viewed as full time participants in continuous interaction with the "professionals" through in person contacts, written reports of progress and problems. Participants should be engaged in a continuing education and training program which is offered by mental health specialists to engender self renewal and to enhance program involvement and commitment.

There is a tendency for a comprehensive system as described here to be used for purposes for which it was never designed. The community and its participants should serve as indicators in accounting for the viability and creditability of this design to ensure that its purpose is realized, namely, to appropriately meet the needs of the chronically mentally ill. There will be need to modify the systems design through extension and modernization, as the community advances in its development to meet the needs of the chronically mentally ill.

VI. SUMMARY

A systems design developmental model is most conducive to meeting the conditions necessary for experimental program planning in comprehensive delivery systems in which there exist a multiplicity of complex needs. A system design offers opportunity to provide guidance and direction to achieve desired results under continuously changing conditions. It is a learning system which is particularly adaptive and responsive to internal and external changes that inevitably arise when the individual, living arrangement and support systems converge and in so doing, produce an interactive process of new patterns and relations. A system design to be purposeful must be monitored and controlled through self-organizing self-regulating and self-modifying system methods and techniques.

REFERENCES

1. For an introduction to the scope, nature and character of the problem see... AFSCME. *Out of Their Beds and Into the Streets: A Report on Deinstitutionalization.* Washington, D.C., American Federation of State, County and Municipal Employees, 1975. De-Jong, G. *The Need for Personal Care Services by Severely Physically Disabled Citizens of Massachusetts.* Report for the Levinson Policy Institute, Brandeis University, 1977. Dickey, J. *Parents Change the System.* DM/MR 28:1., 1978. Elkin, L.A. *Question of Rights,* Project Report of Canadian National Health Grant 608-1000-30, University of Saskatchewan, 1976. Grey, G. "Information Regarding Living Arrangements." Memorandum distributed by United Cerebral Palsy National Office, New York, N.Y., 1978. Wolfensberger, W. *Some Implications for the Principle of Normalization for Architectural Design.* Atlanta: GARC, 1978. Wolfensberger, W. *The Origin and Nature of Our Institutional Models.* Syracuse: Human Policy Press, 1975. Wolfensberger, W. *The Principle of Normalization in Human Services.* Toronto: NIMR, 1972.

2. For discussions on social design building and utilization see... Kilmann, Ralph H. *Social Systems Design.* New York: North Holland, 1977. And De Greene, Kenyon. *Sociotechnical Systems.* Englewood Cliffs, New Jersey: Prentice Hall, Inc. 1973. For a discussion on related designs of inquiry see... Churchman, West C., *The Design of Inquiry*

Systems, New York: Macmillan, 1971, and Rieoken, Henry W. and Boruch, Robert F. (ed.) Social Experimentation. New York: Academic Press, 1974.

3. For a discussion on the use of groups in program planning see...DelBecq, Andre L. and Van de Ven, Andrew H. "A Group Process Model for Problem Identification and Program Planning," Journal of Applied Behavioral Science, (November 1971), 466-92. For a discussion on ideal strategies, see Nadler, Gerald, Work Design, Homewood, Il., Richard D. Irwin, 1970.

4. For references on types of living arrangements see... Belina, V. Planning Your Own Apartment. Belmont, Ca.: Fearon, 1975. Bergman, J. Community Homes for the Retarded. Lexington, Mass.: Lexington Books, 1975. Fanning, J.W. A Common Sense Approach to Community Living Arrangements for the Mentally Retarded. Springfield, Ill.: 1975. Fritz, M. et al. An Apartment Living Plan to Promote Integration and Normalization of Mentally Retarded Adults. Toronto: NIMR, 1971. Goodfellow, R. Group Homes: One Alternative. G. Laurie, 1977. Housing and Home Services for the Disabled. New York: Harper, 1974. NARC. The Right to Choose: Achieving Residential Alternatives in the Community. Arlington, Texas: NARC, 1973. Sipe, H.W. Accounting System for Group Homes for Developmentally Disabled Persons. Eugene: University of Oregon, 1976.

5. See the following references for methods and techniques in "describing complex relations"... Thesen, A., "Some Notes on Systems Models and Modeling", International Journal of Systems Science 5 (1973):145-52. Warfield, John M. "An Assault on Complexity". A Battelle Monograph, N. 3. Columbus, Ohio: Battelle Memorial Institute, 1973. Beckett, John A. Management Dynamics: The New Synthesis. New York: McGraw Hill, 1971.

6. See the following references for "resource availability and analyzing costs"... Irving A. Sirken. "Cost Benefit Analysis: The Technique Its Uses and Limitations", paper prepared for the Economic Development Institute, World Bank, Washington, D.C. Gittinger, J. (ed.) Compounding and Discounting Tables for Project Evaluation, Washington, D.C.: International Bank for Reconstruction and Development, 1973.

7. For a discussion on various models use for design reliability in "deinstitutionalization" see... Heal, L. et. al. "Research on Community Residential Alternatives for the Mentally Retarded." In N.R. Ellis, Ed., International Review of Research in Mental Retardation, Vol. 9, 1978. Knowlton, M. Community Living Arrangements Implementation Package. Harrisburg: 1977. Knowlton, M. "Group Homes." In NARC, 1976 National Forum on Residential Services. Arlington, Texas: NARC, 1976. McGee, J. et al. A Survey of Mentally Retarded Persons Residing in the Community and Nursing Homes. Report available from CASS, University of Nebraska Medical Center, Omaha, Nebraska, 1978. McGee, J. and Hitzing, W. Comprehensive Systems. In NARC, 1976 National Forum on Residential Services. Arlington, Texas: NARC, pp. 13-25, 1976. O'Brien, J. and Poole, C. Planning Spaces: A Manual for Human Services Facilities Development. Atlanta: GARC, 1978.

8. For references on these techniques see... Moder, J.J. Phillips, C.R. Project Management with CPM and P.E.R.T. New York: Rhinhold Publishing, 1964.

9. For a discussion changing patterns in living arrangements see... Roeher, G.A. COM-SERV Canada. In R. Kugel and A. Shearer, eds., Changing Patterns in Residential Services for the Mentally Retarded. (Revised Edition). Washington: PCMR, 1976. Lawrence Kivens and David C. Bolin, "Evaluation in a Community Mental Health Center" in Evaluation, Vol. 3, No. 1-2, 1976.

10. See the following references for community support systems... Office of Evaluation. Metropolitan Placement Unit: Setting a Standard of Quality. First Annual Report, New York: Metropolitan Placement Unit, 1977. Provencal, G. "Foster Families." In NARC, 1976 Residential Services Forum. Arlington, Texas: NARC, pp. 135-155, 1976. Provencal, G. and O. Evans. Resident Manager Education: A Curriculum Model for Educating Foster Parents and Group Home Personnel. St. Clemens, Michigan: McComb-Oakland Regional Center, 1977. Roberts, B. and E. Skarnules. Better Residential Services and How to Pay for Them. Omaha: CASS, 1976.